Low Histamine Cooking

IN YOUR INSTANT POT®

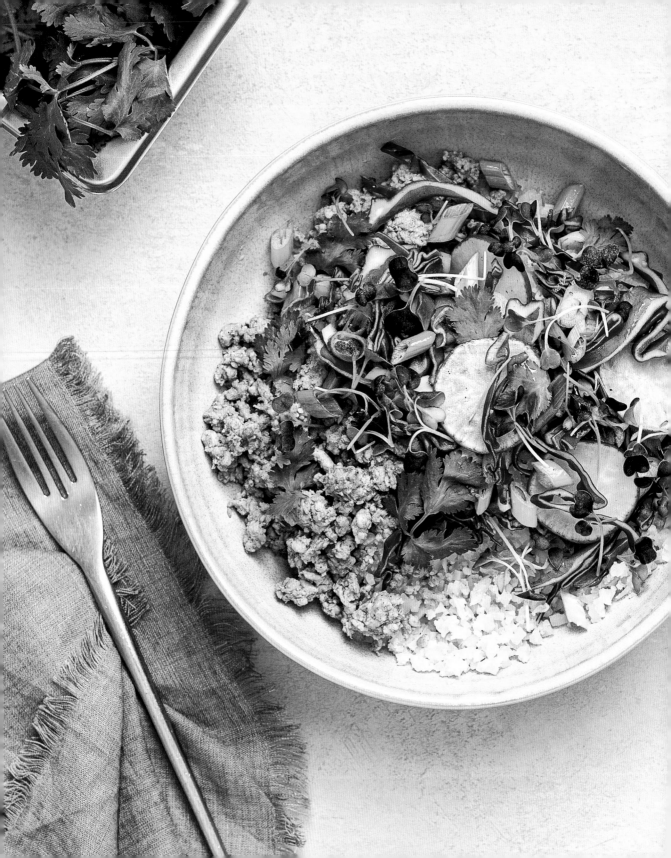

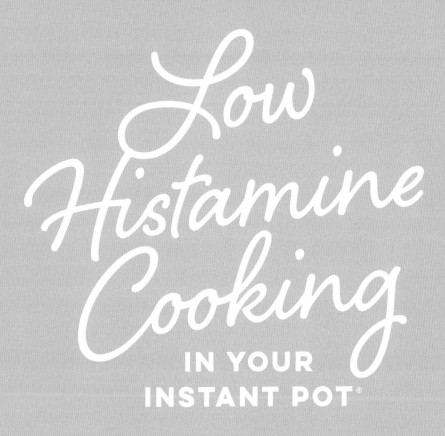

Low Histamine Cooking

IN YOUR
INSTANT POT®

75 Easy Meals
for Everyday Healing

DR. BECKY CAMPBELL

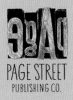

PAGE STREET
PUBLISHING CO.

PAGE STREET
PUBLISHING CO.

First published in 2022 by
Page Street Publishing Co.
27 Congress Street, Suite 1511
Salem, MA 01970
www.pagestreetpublishing.com

Distributed by Macmillan, sales in Canada by The Canadian Manda Group.

26   25   24   23   22   1 2 3 4 5

ISBN-13: 978-1-64567-542-6
ISBN-10: 1-64567-542-4

Library of Congress Control Number: 2021939532

Instant Pot® is a registered trademark of Double Insight, Inc., which was not involved in the creation of this book.

Cover and book design by Meg Baskis for Page Street Publishing Co.

Food Photography by Dani McReynolds
Lifestyle Photography by Lindsey Potter

Printed and bound in the United States

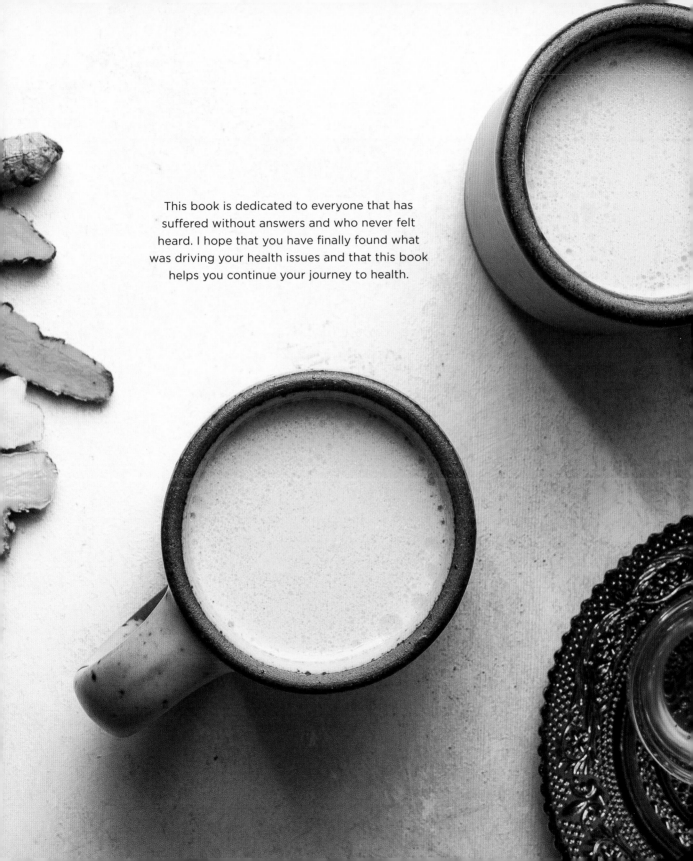

This book is dedicated to everyone that has suffered without answers and who never felt heard. I hope that you have finally found what was driving your health issues and that this book helps you continue your journey to health.

Contents

Introduction:
My Story with Histamine Intolerance   9

One

HISTAMINE INTOLERANCE   11
The Reason You Are Unwell

Histamine What? What Is Histamine
Intolerance?   11

Could This Be You? Symptoms of
Histamine Intolerance   12

But Why? Causes of Histamine Intolerance   15

The Way to Get Well:
Eating a Low Histamine Diet   15

The Yes/No/Maybe List   17

Two

EAT YOURSELF HEALTHY   19
Dr. Becky's Low Histamine
Instant Pot Recipes

Become a Kitchen God(dess): Cooking with
Your Instant Pot   19

Keep It Simple: Instant Pot Food Prep Tips   20

BREAKFAST
Breakfast Hash   22
Asparagus Frittata   25
Savory Sausage Bread Pudding   26
Egg Cups with Mixed Greens   29
Nut and Seed Porridge   30
Soft- or Hard-Boiled Eggs with a Twist   32
Scallion Egg Bites   33
Jumbo Blueberry Pancake   35
Mini Blueberry Loaf   36

LUNCH
Coconut-Poached Chicken   39
Chicken and Creamy Leeks   40
Ground Turkey Taco Bowls   43
The Perfect Pulled Chicken   44
No-Wrap Pork Dumpling   47
Stuffed Bell Peppers   48
Power Veggie Bowl with Carrot-Ginger Dressing   51
Gingery Chicken Salad   52
Almost Niçoise Salad   55
Broccoli Salad   56
Asparagus and Dill Soup   59
Creamy Cauliflower Soup   60
Thai-Style Carrot Soup   63

Parsnip Soup 64

Chicken Zoodle Soup 67

Green Minestrone 68

Sweet Potato Chowder 69

DINNER

Garlic Butter Chicken 70

Lamb Shank with Shallots 73

Tortilla-less Green Chicken Enchiladas 74

Sausage and Kale Stew 77

Easy Beef Stew with Carrot and Sweet Potato 78

Pork Chops with Cherry Sauce 81

Whole Chicken with Pearl Onions 82

Sweet Potato Shepherd's Pie 85

Pork and Collard Greens 86

Braised Short Ribs with Gravy 89

Melt-in-Your-Mouth Carnitas 90

Hearty Pot Roast 93

Stuffed Cabbage Soup 94

Quick Beef Pho 97

Healing Chicken Soup with Ginger and Turmeric 98

Root Vegetable Soup 101

SIDES

Glazed Carrots 102

Fondant Potatoes 105

Braised Kale 106

Coconut Cauliflower Rice 107

Honey Beets 108

Mashed Sweet Potatoes 111

Garlic Mashed Cauliflower 112

Mini Cauliflower Patties 115

Sesame Cabbage 116

Steamed Artichokes with Garlic Butter 119

Brown Butter Asparagus 120

Zoodles with Herb Butter 123

Zucchini Medallions 124

Whole Herby Cauliflower 125

Steamed Sweet Potato 126

SNACKS

Cauliflower Hummus 129

Large Batch Golden Turmeric Milk 130

Coconut Chia Pudding 133

Sunflower Seed Queso 134

Anti-Inflammatory Egg Salad 137

Antihistamine Artichoke Dip 138

Caramelized Onion Dip 141

DESSERT

Crustless Sweet Potato Pie 142

Upside-Down Apple Cake 145

Chunky Apple Compote 146

Maple Blondies 149

Coconut Custard 150

Soothing Tapioca Pudding 153

Sticky Ginger Pudding 154

Mixed Berry Compote 157

Blueberry Cobbler 158

Cherry Apple Crumble 161

References 162

Acknowledgments 162

About the Author 163

Index 164

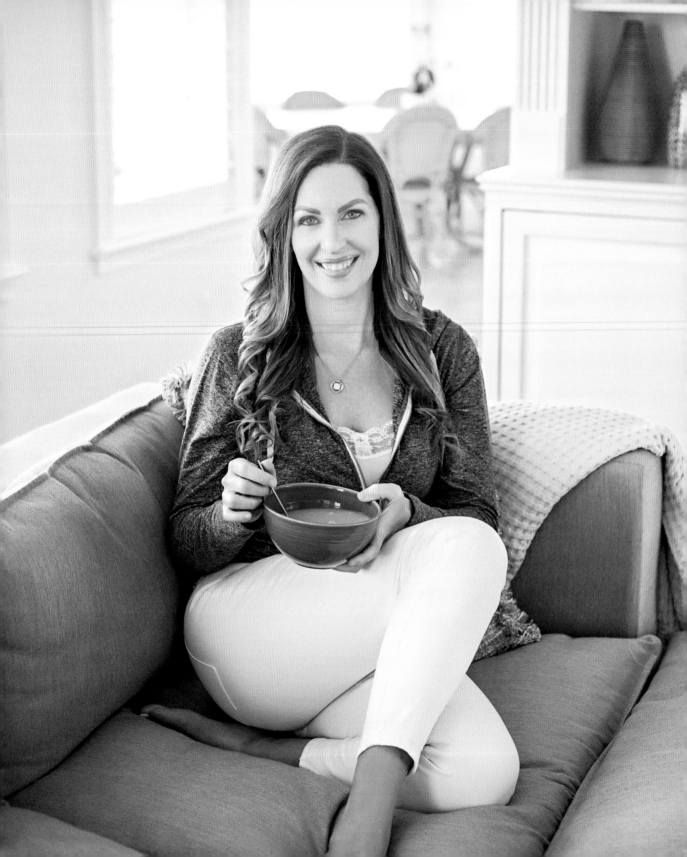

INTRODUCTION:

My Story with Histamine Intolerance

If you've read my other books, *The 4-Phase Histamine Reset Plan* and *The 30-Day Thyroid Reset Plan*, or follow my blog or social media, you already know a bit about my story. You know that healing histamine intolerance is just as personal to me as it may be to you.

For years, I suffered from undiagnosed thyroid issues that were driven by gut problems, viral infections and heavy metals. I was lucky enough to work with a functional medicine doctor and get diagnosed with Hashimoto's disease. I overcame my thyroid issues and regained much of my health naturally, but some symptoms remained and kept affecting my well-being. I was experiencing strange symptoms that included migraines, skin conditions, anxiety and panic attacks, heart palpitations, tingling of my scalp and so on.

It wasn't until years after my initial thyroid diagnosis that I learned about histamine intolerance as a functional medicine practitioner. I finally started to piece together the puzzle of my health. It turns out my mysterious symptoms were driven by mast cell activation syndrome (MCAS) and therefore, histamine intolerance.

This diagnosis was life changing. I finally knew what to do and learned how to improve my health. I began following the low histamine plan I outlined in *The 4-Phase Histamine Reset Plan*. I was able to recover my body, eliminate my symptoms and live a healthy day-to-day life. I decided to dedicate my practice to histamine intolerance, a lesser-known yet common health condition.

I am going to be honest, though. Figuring out how to cook following a low histamine diet was challenging at first. I love food and there was no way I was going to eat a bland or boring diet. This challenge took me on an exciting new culinary journey. I recreated my favorite recipes and created new delicious ones—all with low histamine ingredients.

Using my Instant Pot® was a life saver. The Instant Pot helps prevent histamine buildup and keep histamine levels low in your meals. I genuinely believe that everyone should learn how to cook with an Instant Pot. So, I dedicated this entire cookbook to my favorite Instant Pot recipes to support your recovery from histamine intolerance and keep you healthy and energized.

See you in the kitchen. Let's get cooking,

Dr. Becky Campbell

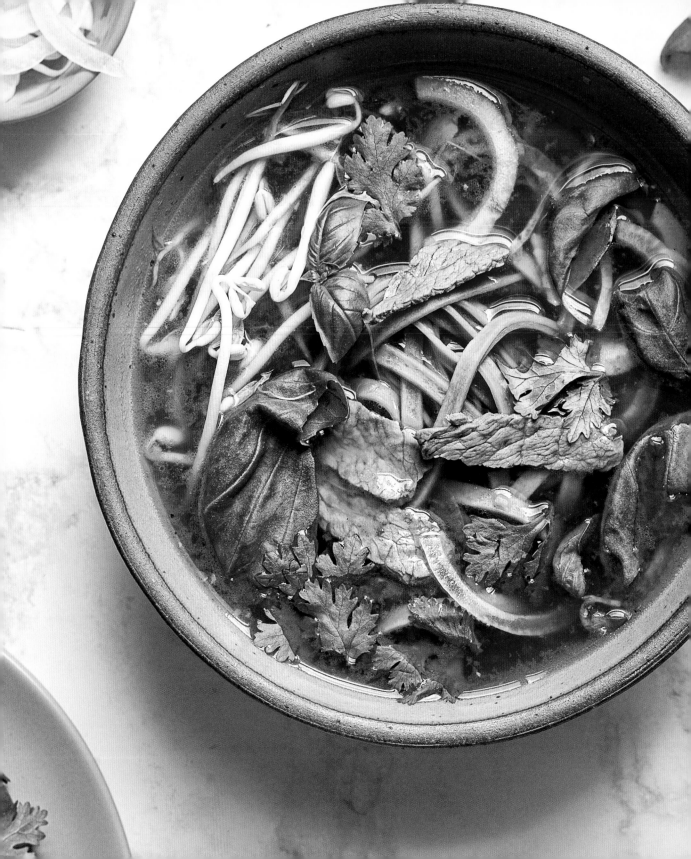

One
HISTAMINE INTOLERANCE

The Reason You Are Unwell

Histamine What? What Is Histamine Intolerance?

Before we jump into histamine intolerance, you need to understand what histamine is and how it can turn into a problem. Histamine is a naturally occurring chemical in your body. It often gets a bad rap because of antihistamine medications for allergies.

Histamine is far from bad, though. It is an essential part of your immune system and plays a number of important roles in your body.

Histamine's primary role is to help your body get rid of allergens. When foreign invaders such as allergens or toxins attack your body, your body immediately sends an army of chemical messengers to alert your immune system. Histamine is one of these crucial chemicals. With the help of histamine, your white blood cells can rush in to kill pathogens. This response, however, results in allergic reactions that prompt many people to reach for antihistamines for relief from allergy symptoms.

Most people don't know that histamine supports your digestion. It does this by releasing hydro-chloric acid to help break down your food and bacteria, preventing bacteria buildup in your gut. Histamine also plays a significant role in your nervous system and brain. It serves as a neurotransmitter delivering messages between your brain and your body.

You see, histamine is not the problem. When your body has just enough histamine to take care of allergens and other pathogens, it is a wonderful protective mechanism. The problem arises when your body has too much histamine.

Histamine intolerance is not sensitivity to hista-mine, as you might imagine hearing the term. It's a problem having to do with histamine buildup. When your body releases too much histamine and/or is unable to break down excess histamine after it's done doing its job, histamine buildup occurs.

Under normal circumstances, in a healthy body, your body sends enzymes to break down hista-mine. One of these enzymes is the diamine oxidase (DAO) enzyme that does the majority of histamine cleanup and supports a proper hista-mine balance. Another one is histamine N-methyltransferase (HNMT), which helps mop up excess histamine in the spaces between cells around your spine, liver, kidneys and lungs.

When your body has too much histamine, however, it becomes difficult for your body to break down and metabolize the excess. This will result in hista-mine buildup known as histamine intolerance. Histamine intolerance can affect your entire body, including your gut, brain, cardiovascular system, lungs and skin. It can lead to a list of unwanted and uncomfortable symptoms that can interfere with your quality of life and overall well-being.

Could This Be You? Symptoms of Histamine Intolerance

Symptoms of histamine intolerance may be different for everyone. For many people, they are quite similar to seasonal allergies. For others, symptoms may be more severe. Symptoms may vary from mild to debilitating. You may only experience a few random mild symptoms, or you may recognize every single one from this list.

Symptoms of histamine intolerance include:

- Itchy skin, eyes, ears and nose
- Eczema or other types of dermatitis
- Hives
- Red eyes
- Facial swelling
- Congestion or runny nose
- Seasonal allergies
- Asthma
- Tightness in the throat
- Crawling sensation on the skin or the scalp
- Difficulty regulating body temperature
- A sudden drop in blood pressure when standing up
- Low blood pressure
- Fast heart rate
- Heart palpitations
- Dizziness or vertigo
- Difficulty falling asleep or sleep issues
- Fatigue
- Confusion
- Brain fog
- Irritability
- Anxiety or panic attacks
- Migraines and headaches
- Acid reflux
- Diarrhea
- Digestive discomfort
- Dermatographia (skin drawing)
- Abnormal menstrual cycle
- Premenstrual syndrome (PMS)

Symptoms of Histamine Intolerance

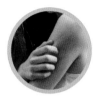

ITCHY SKIN, EYES, EARS, AND NOSE

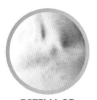

ECZEMA OR OTHER TYPES OF DERMATITIS

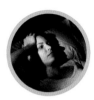

DIFFICULTY FALLING ASLEEP OR SLEEP ISSUES

CRAWLING SENSATION ON THE SKIN OR THE SCALP

DIFFICULTY REGULATING BODY TEMPERATURE

DIZZINESS WHEN STANDING UP

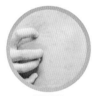

HIVES

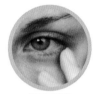

RED EYES

FACIAL SWELLING

SEASONAL ALLERGIES

ASTHMA

CONGESTION OR RUNNY NOSE

LOW BLOOD PRESSURE

FAST HEART RATE

HEART PALPITATIONS

DIZZINESS OR VERTIGO

TIGHTNESS IN THE THROAT

FATIGUE

CONFUSION

BRAIN FOG

IRRITABILITY

ANXIETY OR PANIC ATTACKS

MIGRAINES AND HEADACHES

ACID REFLUX

DIARRHEA

DIGESTIVE DISCOMFORT

DERMATOGRAPHIA (SKIN DRAWING)

ABNORMAL MENSTRUAL CYCLE

PREMENSTRUAL SYNDROME (PMS)

Main Causes of Histamine Intolerance

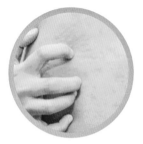

MAST CELL ACTIVATION SYNDROME (MCAS)

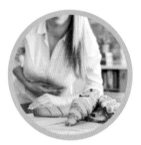

GLUTEN INTOLERANCE

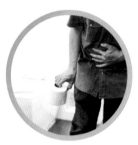

LEAKY GUT SYNDROME

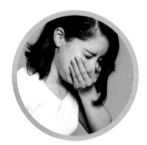

GUT INFECTIONS

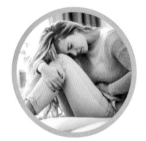

INFLAMMATORY DIGESTIVE DISEASES

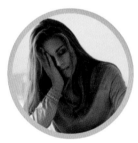

NUTRIENT DEFICIENCIES

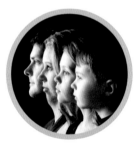

GENETIC MUTATIONS

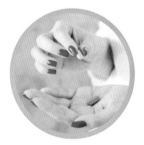

CERTAIN MEDICATIONS

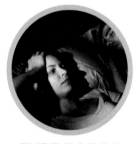

EMF EXPOSURE

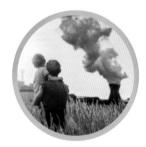

ENVIRONMENTAL TOXINS
INCLUDING MOLD, AIR POLLUTION,
PESTICIDES, MERCURY,
AND VARIOUS CHEMICALS

But Why? Causes of Histamine Intolerance

In my book, *The 4-Phase Histamine Reset Plan*, I discuss the underlying factors that may lead to histamine intolerance. Some of these factors decrease DAO enzyme functions, while others affect the amount of histamine that gets released into your body.

The underlying causes of histamine intolerance may include:

- Mast cell activation syndrome (MCAS)
- Gluten intolerance
- Leaky gut syndrome
- Gut infections
- Inflammatory digestive diseases
- Nutrient deficiencies
- Genetic mutations
- Certain medications
- Electric and magnetic field (EMF) exposure
- Environmental toxins including mold, air pollution, pesticides, mercury and various chemicals

You may be affected by one, two or all of these underlying causes of histamine intolerance. If you are experiencing symptoms of histamine intolerance, I highly recommend that you work with a functional medicine doctor well versed in histamine intolerance rather than doing the guesswork by yourself at home.

Uncovering the root causes of your health issues can help you manage your condition and improve your health. My team and I have worked with thousands of people like you. Don't hesitate to make an appointment at drbeckycampbell.com.

The Way to Get Well: Eating a Low Histamine Diet

If you have histamine intolerance or suspect that you do, then it is critical that you reduce your histamine bucket. The first and most crucial step in reducing your histamine load is following a low histamine diet.

In my book, *The 4-Phase Histamine Reset Plan*, I outlined a 4-phase low histamine plan to reduce your histamine bucket and improve your symptoms. If you are experiencing symptoms of histamine intolerance, I highly recommend following this protocol. If you have already completed your 4-phase histamine reset, I still recommend that you follow a mostly low histamine diet.

So why is eating a low histamine diet so important? If you have histamine intolerance, your body is overloaded with histamine. No matter how hard it's trying, it cannot break down all the excess histamine. A diet full of high histamine foods only adds fuel to the fire and makes it impossible for your body to recover.

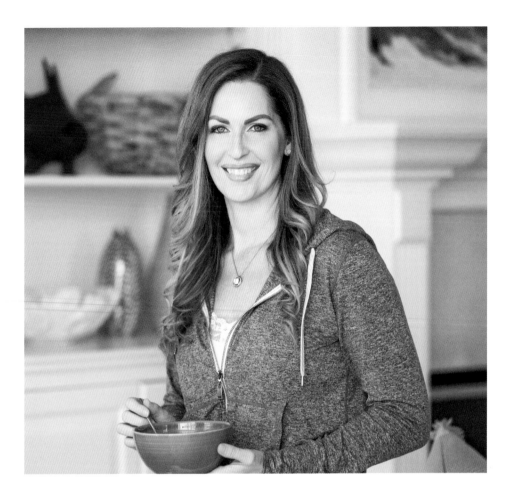

Following a low histamine diet, on the other hand, helps to reduce your daily histamine load. It allows your body to have a breather, break down excess histamine and finally repair and recover. It is an anti-inflammatory and nutrient-dense diet that supports and nourishes your body. Don't worry, it is not a bland diet, either. Once you try my low histamine Instant Pot recipes, you will find that a low histamine diet is delicious and nutritious at the same time. Trust me, even your family and friends will love it. I have made a list of Yes (eat freely), No (completely avoid) and Maybe (try to eat them and see how you feel) foods. Most of the foods are there in relation to histamine, but remember that histamine causes inflammation. I also want you to keep foods that cause inflammation out like gluten, conventional dairy, processed sugar, legumes and grains. This is all reflected in the list to the right.

Dr. Becky's Low Histamine Plan

PHASE 1

THE YES / NO / MAYBE LIST

YES FOODS (EAT FREELY)

PROTEIN
(must be fresh or frozen)

Beef
Bison
Chicken
Duck
Elk
Lamb
Pasture-Raised Eggs
(whites must be cooked)
Pheasant
Pork
Rabbit
Seafood
(must be very fresh)
Turkey
Venison
Wild Boar

FRUITS
(must be fresh or frozen)

Apples
Apricots
Blackberries
Blueberries
Cherries
Exotic fruit
(star fruit, quince)
Grapes
Melon
Pears

VEGETABLES

Anise/Fennel Root
Artichoke
Arugula
Asparagus
Beets
Bell Peppers
Bok Choy
Broccoli
Brussels Sprouts
Cabbage
Carrots
Cauliflower
Celery
Collard Greens
Cucumber
Garlic
Green Beans
Greens
(beet, mustard, turnip)
Jicama
Kale
Leeks
Lettuce
(bibb, butter, red)
Onion/Shallot
Parsnips
Rutabaga
Sweet Potatoes/Yams
Swiss Chard
Turnip
Watercress
Zucchini
Any other veggies not listed
in the no or maybe list

FATS

Extra Virgin Olive Oil
Ghee
Grass-Fed Butter
Coconut Oil

SWEETENER

Black Strap Molasses
Honey *(local is best)*
Maple Syrup/Maple Sugar
Coconut Sugar

FLOURS

Arrowroot
Cassava
Tapioca
Coconut Flour

OTHERS

Celtic or Himalayan Sea Salt
Leafy Herbs
Pepper
White Tea and Herbal Teas
Coconut Products
*(coconut milk, coconut
butter, shredded coconut)*
Any spices that are not on
the no list

NO FOODS (DO NOT EAT)

PROTEIN

Anything that is in the
Yes Protein List that is
not fresh and/or leftovers

FRUITS

Avocado
Citrus
Dried Fruit
(apricots, prunes, dates, figs, raisins)
Strawberries
Tomato
Banana

VEGETABLES

Eggplant
Spinach

VINEGARS

All Vinegars
*(except gluten-free distilled white
vinegar and apple cider vinegar, which
are the lowest in histamine)*
Vinegar-Containing
Products
(e.g. olives, mustard, ketchup, mayo)

NUTS
(highest in histamine)

Cashews
Walnuts

ADDITIONAL FOODS
*(not all high in histamine but
may cause inflammation)*

Alcohol *(especially red wine)*
Beans
Chocolate
Cinnamon
Dairy
Fermented Foods
Gluten
Grains
Peanuts
Soy

SPICES

Anise
Cinnamon
Cloves
Curry Powder
Paprika/Cayenne
Nutmeg
Seasoning packets with
restrictive ingredients
Food labeled "with spices"

MAYBE LIST
(EAT MODERATELY)

FRUITS

Raspberries
Kiwi
Lemon
Lime
Mango
Nectarine
Papaya
Peach
Plum

VEGETABLES

Mushrooms
Peas
Pumpkin
Squash

NUTS

Soaked Almonds
Pecans
Pistachio
Soaked Brazil & Pine Nuts

FLOUR
*(Most people do ok with these
but check your tolerance)*

Almond Flour

SEED & SEED BUTTERS

Flax
Sesame/Tahini
Sunflower
Pumpkin

OTHER

Apple Cider Vinegar
Dried Herbs/Spices
Gelatin/Collagen
Gluten-Free Distilled
White Vinegar Yeast

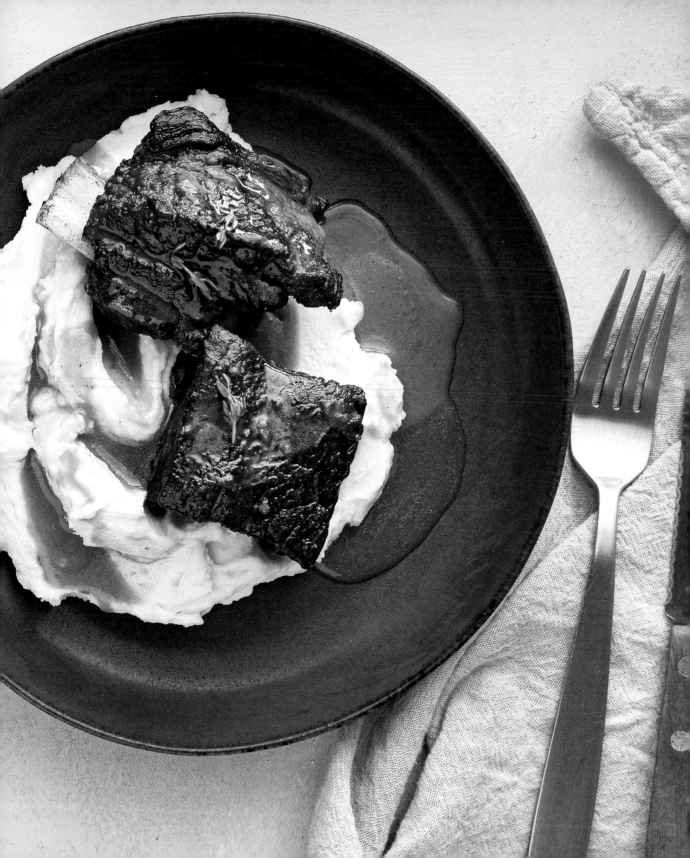

Two

EAT YOURSELF HEALTHY

Dr. Becky's Low Histamine Instant Pot Recipes

Become a Kitchen God(dess): Cooking with Your Instant Pot

I love cooking with my Instant Pot for so many reasons. One of these reasons, of course, is practicality. Let's be honest. I am a busy mother, doctor and business owner. I don't have time to spend five hours in the kitchen. The Instant Pot cuts down on both cooking and cleanup time. You can use your Instant Pot for just about anything, from broths to soups, sautés, stews, vegetables and even hard-boiled eggs. If you are a busy person like me, you will love it.

Even better, the Instant Pot is perfect for people with histamine intolerance. It's a cooking method made just for you! Because the Instant Pot reduces cooking time, it also decreases the chance of histamine buildup. This is particularly true if you are cooking meat. Using an Instant Pot is a great way to make delicious low histamine bone broth. Instead of simmering it for 24 hours, you can make bone broth within 2 hours and then freeze it right away, which significantly decreases the amount of histamine.

In my book, *The 4-Phase Histamine Reset Plan*, I share some delicious low histamine recipes. Ever since its release, I've been getting requests to share more recipes, and it's finally time. I've dedicated this entire book to my favorite low histamine Instant Pot recipes.

Keep It Simple: Instant Pot Food Prep Tips

You are a busy person. I get it. Using an Instant Pot reduces cooking time, but how to reduce prep time? Here are some great tips:

MAKE A MEAL PLAN

Instead of thinking about what to eat for lunch during breakfast or what to cook for dinner when you get home, make a meal plan for the entire week or even the entire month. A weekly or monthly meal plan can save so much time. It can make grocery shopping and cooking so much easier.

SHOP ACCORDING TO YOUR NEEDS

Never go to the grocery store without a plan or when you are hungry. You will be tempted to buy some unhealthy, high histamine options and you will likely spend more money too. Whether you like grocery shopping once a week or a couple of times a week, always bring a list based on your meal plan.

MORE SHOPPING TIPS

Shop organic to avoid pesticides, herbicides, hormones and chemicals. Choose grass-fed beef, pork and lamb, pasture-raised poultry and eggs, wild-caught fish and wild game for animal protein. Grow your own vegetables or join a Community Supported Agriculture (CSA) group. Buy in season and buy local. To reduce costs, buy frozen if needed, shop in bulk and watch out for sales and coupons.

WASH AND PREP AHEAD OF TIME

When you get home from the farmer's market or grocery store, wash your produce right away. Portion them out before you store them in your fridge or freezer. If you do this, you can just grab them when you need them. I recommend that you make your own fruit and veggie wash with water and vinegar.

COOK IN MULTIPLE BATCHES

Meal planning and cooking more than one batch saves a lot of time. When you are making a recipe, you can cook multiple batches. Freeze what you don't need right away and save them for another day.

PREP YOUR SALADS AND CHIA PUDDING IN A CANNING JAR

Using a canning jar for your salad is a super simple, smart and fun idea. You can prepare your salad the night before as a convenient, on-the-go and ready-to-eat lunch. You can also prepare your chia pudding the night before for a ready-to-eat breakfast.

PREP YOUR SNACKS

Choosing healthy snacks is one of the toughest things for many people. If you don't plan your snacks ahead of time, you may be more tempted to reach for less healthy options. Prep your snacks ahead of time and you'll always have something fresh or homemade available with you. Having some fruits or veggie sticks around to dip into your Cauliflower Hummus (page 129) or Sunflower Seed Queso (page 134) is a great idea.

A WORD ON LEFTOVERS

Many individuals with histamine intolerance experience symptoms when eating leftover foods. I recommend freezing your food immediately after you prepare it. By freezing your food, you can meal plan and cook ahead for the week. There are also foods that you can prepare and store for a few days in your fridge.

Not everyone reacts negatively to leftovers though. If you are not sensitive to leftover foods, you can warm and serve leftover vegetables from the night before. I don't recommend using leftover meat, though. Experiment with what feels good for your body.

CHICKEN TENDERLOINS

I recommend buying a package of chicken tenderloins. Divide them up and put them in freezer bags, with two to three tenderloins per bag. Keep them in your freezer until you need them. They are super easy to defrost in the morning and you can use them in your lunch.

FROZEN PATTIES

I recommend buying ground chicken, turkey, grass-fed beef, bison or lamb and making patties from them to freeze, so that you can just pull them out when you need them. This saves some prep time while keeping your diet low histamine.

PORTION YOUR VEGGIES

Portioning your vegetables ahead of time saves so much prep time. You can portion your raw veggies in bags and use them for salads later. You can also portion out your precooked vegetables in bags for future use.

COLLARD GREEN WRAPS

You can make your collard green wraps ahead of time. Store them in your fridge and use them as needed throughout the week.

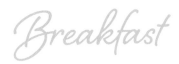

Breakfast

Breakfast is the most important meal of the day. A nourishing, low histamine breakfast will set you up for a symptom-free, energized day. It will also motivate you to follow your low histamine protocol for the rest of the day. These low histamine Instant Pot breakfast recipes require minimal prep and fuss. They are simple and perfect to start your busy day and yet they also work for a slow-paced family breakfast on the weekends. I love savory breakfasts and am always down for a good Asparagus Frittata (page 25) or Breakfast Hash (below). On a busy day, the Nut and Seed Porridge (page 30) is my favorite go-to.

BREAKFAST HASH

Breakfast hash is a classic, except this one is healthy, nourishing, nutrient-dense, fiber-powered and low histamine. It's loaded with histamine-lowering quercetin-rich vegetables and herbs, including onions, bell peppers, oregano and salt. It's a perfect choice to share with your family.

Yield: 3-4 SERVINGS

3 bell peppers of assorted colors

1 onion, red or white

1 large sweet potato

1 tbsp (15 ml) olive oil

½ tsp oregano

½ tsp salt

¼ tsp pepper

½ cup (120 ml) chicken or vegetable broth

3–4 eggs, for serving

2–3 small radishes, sliced thin, for garnish

2 tbsp (10 g) chopped chives, for garnish

Cut the bell peppers, onion and sweet potato into similar size pieces, about 1½ inches (4 cm) in size. Place them in a medium bowl and toss with the olive oil, oregano, salt and pepper. Transfer them to the Instant Pot and pour in the broth.

Seal the Instant Pot lid and set it to cook with high pressure for 3 minutes. Quick release the pressure and serve with eggs cooked to your liking. Top with radish and chives, and enjoy.

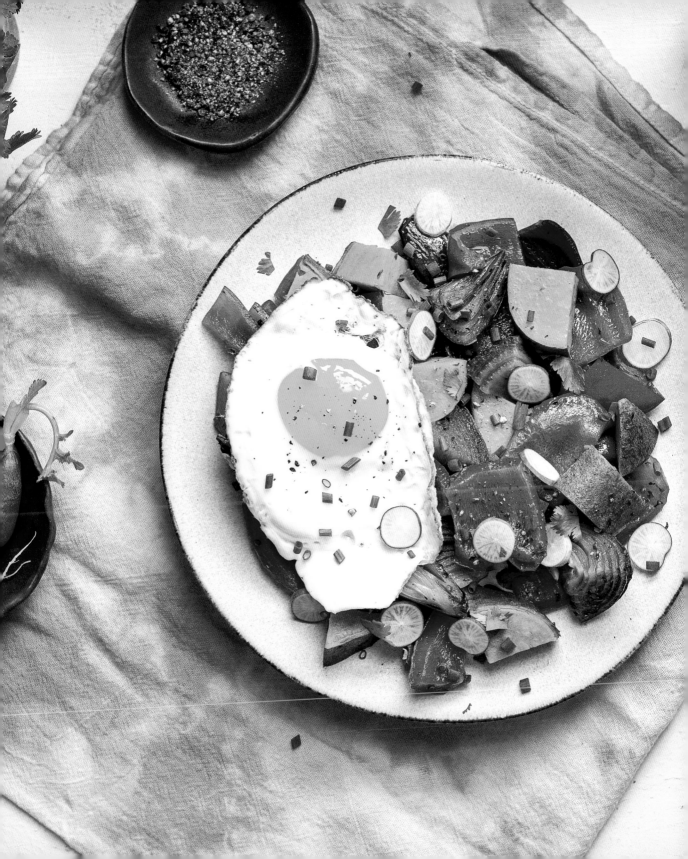

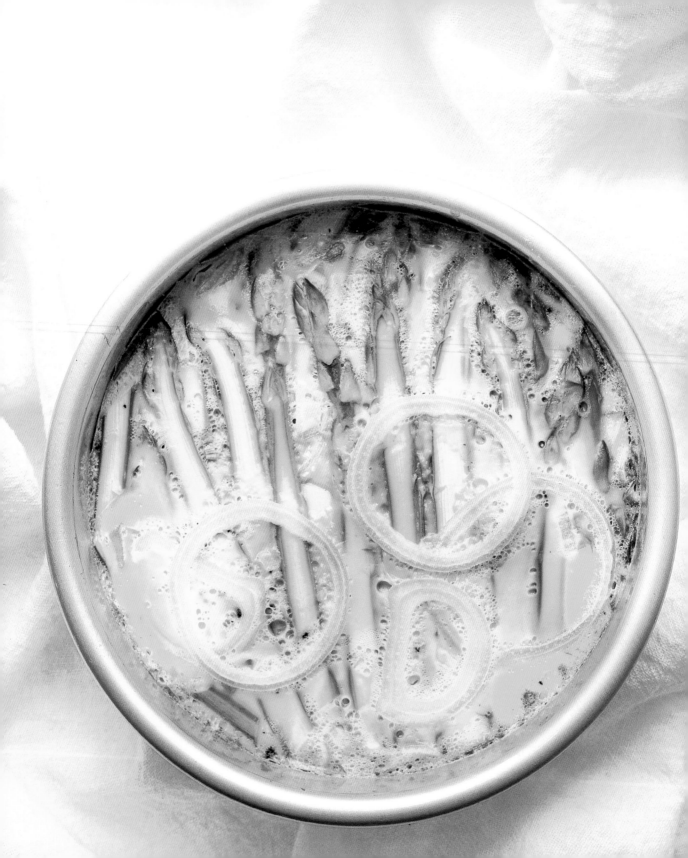

ASPARAGUS FRITTATA

Choosing a frittata for breakfast is another great way to sneak in some veggies at breakfast time. Asparagus is anti-inflammatory and low in histamine. It's a balanced choice with plenty of protein, antioxidants and minerals to keep you satisfied and energized.

Yield: 4 SERVINGS

4–5 asparagus stalks

6 eggs

½ tsp salt

¼ tsp pepper

½ shallot, thinly sliced

2 tsp (10 ml) vegetable oil

1 cup (240 ml) water

Thinly slice the asparagus. Reserve four to five pieces to arrange on top of the frittata and cut the remaining stalks into ½-inch (1.3-cm) pieces.

In a medium bowl, whisk the eggs with the salt and pepper. Mix in the smaller asparagus pieces and most of the shallot—reserve a couple of pieces for the top, if desired. Rub the vegetable oil around the sides and bottom of a 6-inch (15-cm) pan. Pour the egg mixture in and arrange the reserved asparagus and shallots on top. Cover it with foil and place on the trivet inside of the Instant Pot with 1 cup (240 ml) of water in the bottom.

Cook with high pressure for 6 minutes, then slow release for 10 minutes, open the quick release valve and remove the lid. These frittatas can be served warm or at room temperature.

SAVORY SAUSAGE BREAD PUDDING

If you love savory breakfasts as much as I do, you will love this savory sausage bread pudding. Make it with store-bought Paleo bread for a gluten-free hearty meal. It's also a delicious low histamine option.

Yield: 3–4 SERVINGS

2 cups (86 g) or 5 slices Paleo bread

½ lb (226 g) turkey sausage

2 tbsp (30 ml) olive oil

1 onion, halved and sliced

½ tsp + a pinch of salt, divided

½ bunch Swiss chard, stems removed and sliced into ½-inch (1.3-cm) pieces

2 eggs

½ cup (120 ml) coconut milk

¼ tsp pepper

1 tbsp (3 g) chives, finely chopped

1 tbsp (4 g) fresh parsley, finely chopped

1 cup (240 ml) water

Cut the Paleo bread into ½-inch (1.3-cm) pieces and then leave them out for 1 to 2 days to harden, or toast them in the oven at 300°F (149°C) for 10 to 20 minutes, until they are thoroughly dried out. This step can be done ahead of time.

Break the sausage into 1-inch (2.5-cm) pieces. Turn the Instant Pot on to the sauté setting and heat the olive oil. Sear the sausage pieces until browned on each side, 3 to 5 minutes per side, and then remove them from the Instant Pot and set aside. Without cleaning the Instant Pot, add in the onion with a pinch of salt and cook until just beginning to soften, about 3 minutes. Add the Swiss chard and cook for an additional 1 to 2 minutes, until wilted. Transfer to the bowl with the sausage and add the toasted bread.

In a separate bowl, whisk together the eggs, coconut milk, ½ teaspoon of salt, pepper, chives and parsley. Pour the egg mixture over the other ingredients and stir well to coat. Allow everything to sit for 10 minutes, stirring occasionally to allow the bread to soak up the egg mixture.

Transfer the bread pudding to a 6- or 8-inch (15- or 20-cm) baking dish that will fit into your Instant Pot. Cover with foil and place on the trivet inside of the Instant Pot with 1 cup (240 ml) of water in the base. Seal the lid and set to cook with high pressure for 25 minutes. Quick release the pressure and then remove the foil. Allow the steam to evaporate for 5 to 10 minutes before serving.

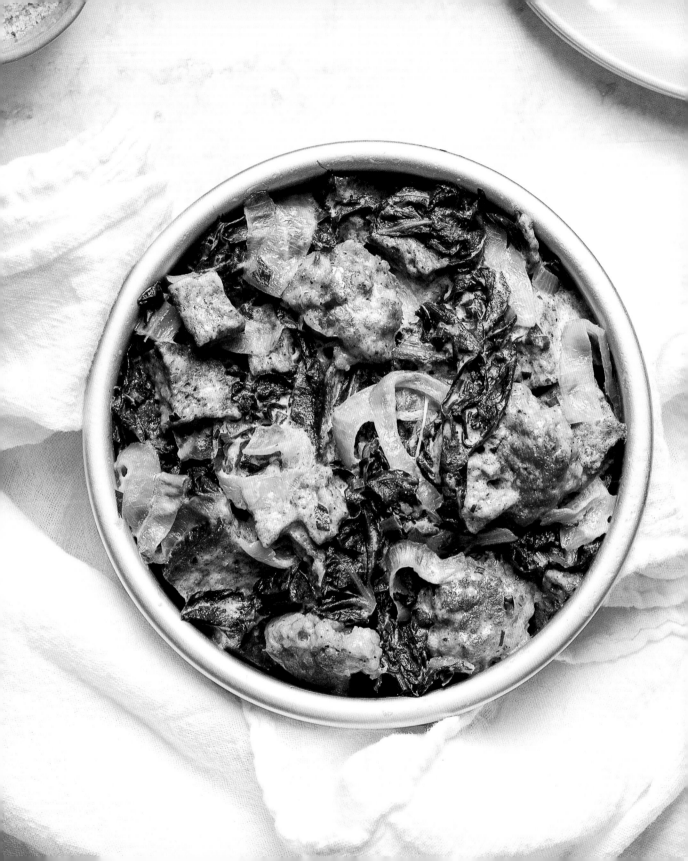

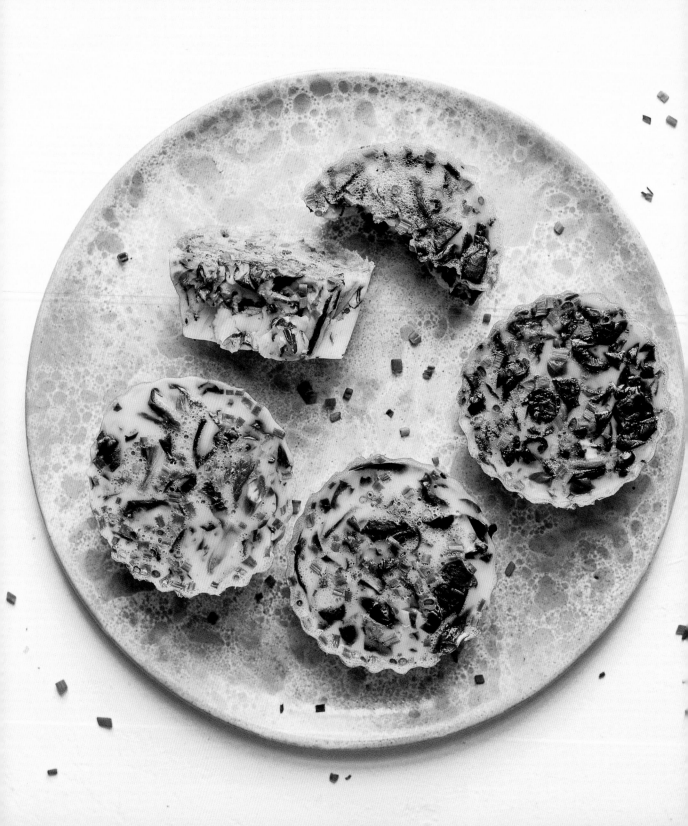

EGG CUPS WITH MIXED GREENS

Most people don't include any vegetables in their breakfast, but adding some chopped greens to this recipe will boost your energy and brainpower to get you going in the morning. The protein from the eggs will keep you satisfied until lunchtime.

Yield: 5-6 SERVINGS

2 tbsp (30 ml) olive oil

¼ cup (17 g) roughly chopped greens such as kale, mustard greens or Swiss chard

5 eggs

¼ tsp salt

¼ tsp pepper

2 tbsp (6 g) chives or other fresh herb

1 cup (240 ml) water

Turn the Instant Pot onto the sauté function and heat the olive oil. Add the greens and cook for 2 to 3 minutes, tossing often, until the greens are wilted. Remove them from the heat and allow to cool slightly.

In a bowl, whisk together the eggs, salt and pepper. Add in the chives and cooked greens, and mix well to combine all the ingredients.

Fill five to six muffin cups three-quarters full and cover them with a silicone lid or foil. Pour 1 cup (240 ml) of water into the Instant Pot and place the trivet inside, then carefully place the muffin cups on top of the trivet. Close the lid and seal the valve. Cook with high pressure for 7 minutes. Allow them to cool for 5 minutes before carefully opening the quick release valve.

NUT AND SEED PORRIDGE

I have some great news! You can eat porridge on a low histamine diet. The nuts and seeds in this breakfast porridge are abundant with antioxidants and anti-inflammatory benefits. Pair it with your favorite berries and you are good to go.

Yield: 3-4 SERVINGS

1¼ cups (300 ml) coconut milk

3 tbsp (30 g) chia seeds (for thick porridge add another 1 tbsp [10 g] of chia)

¼ cup (34 g) sunflower seeds

¼ cup (35 g) pumpkin seeds (if not tolerated, replace with sunflower seeds)

1 tbsp (9 g) sesame seeds

1 tbsp (15 ml) honey

¼ tsp salt

Place the coconut milk, chia seeds, sunflower seeds, pumpkin seeds, sesame seeds, honey and salt in the Instant Pot and stir to combine. Use the porridge setting to cook with low pressure for 10 minutes. Allow to naturally cool for 10 minutes before releasing the steam valve. Serve with your favorite fresh or frozen fruits.

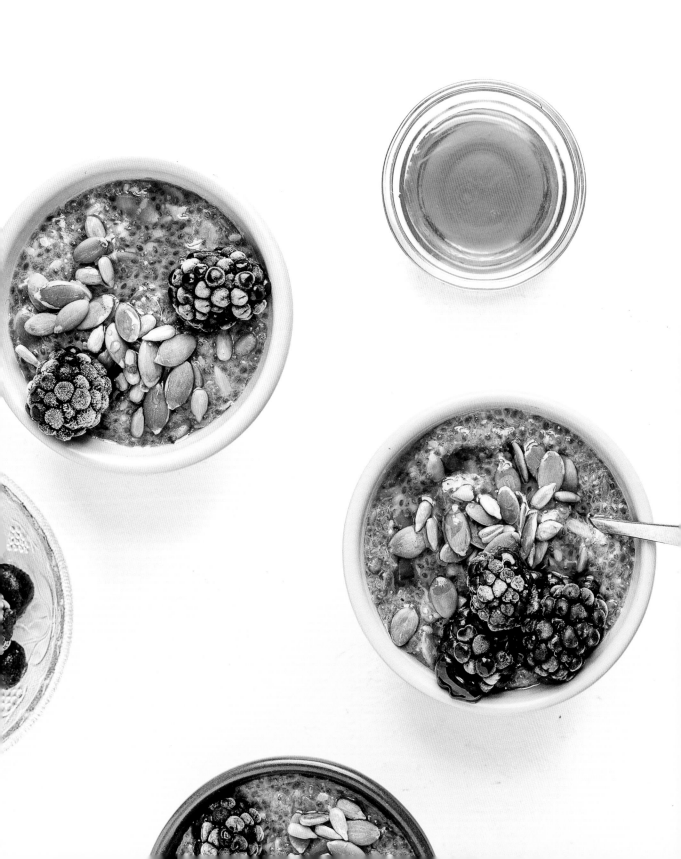

SOFT– OR HARD–BOILED EGGS WITH A TWIST

It cannot get easier than this. High-quality protein, anti-inflammatory omega-3 fatty acids and brain-protecting B vitamins. What else do you need? It's simple, low histamine and satisfying.

1 cup (240 ml) water

Eggs

Pour 1 cup (240 ml) of water into the Instant Pot and place the trivet inside. Carefully lay as many eggs as you'd like onto the trivet and seal the Instant Pot lid.

For a very soft yolk, set the timer for 3 minutes at high pressure. Once it beeps, quick release the pressure and transfer the eggs to an ice bath or run under cold water. Increase the cooking time for firmer eggs. Seven minutes will result in a fully hard-boiled egg, while 5 minutes will have a mostly set yolk that is slightly jammy in the center.

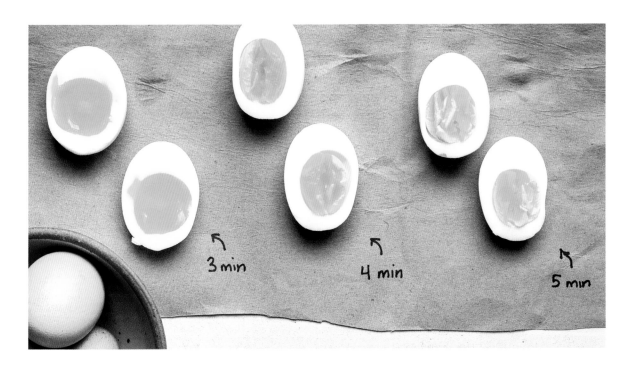

SCALLION EGG BITES

I wasn't lying when I said that there are endless ways to make eggs. Scallions are rich in nutrients and low in histamine. These scallion egg bites are perfect as a sit-down meal or an on-the-go option.

Yield: 6 SERVINGS

4 eggs

½ tsp salt

¼ tsp pepper

3–4 scallions, sliced

1 cup (240 ml) water

In a medium bowl, whisk the eggs, salt and pepper. Add in the scallions and incorporate them into the mixture.

Divide the egg mixture between six miniature muffin molds. Place them on the trivet inside the Instant Pot and carefully pour 1 cup (240 ml) of water into the bottom of the pot. Seal the lid and set the time for 7 minutes with high pressure. Once finished, quick release the pressure and remove the egg bites from their molds.

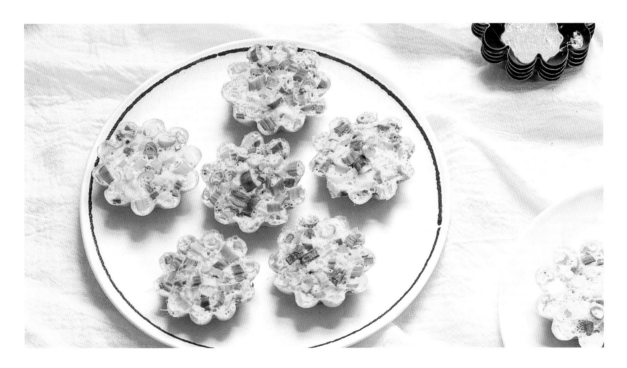

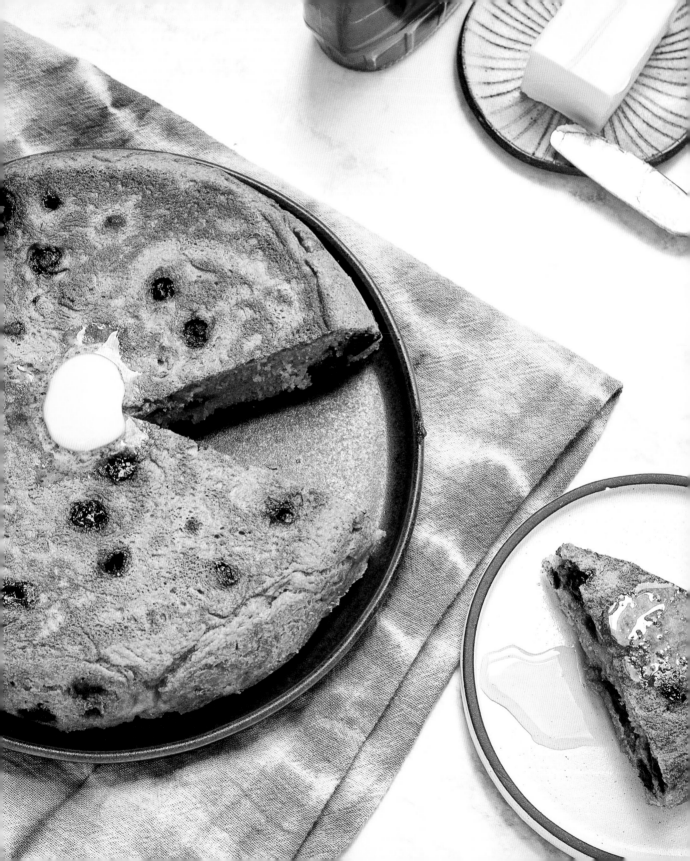

JUMBO BLUEBERRY PANCAKE

This is a classic breakfast recipe healthified just for you. It's perfect for Sunday brunch, but you can enjoy it any day of the week. The blueberries are rich in quercetin, which helps lower your histamine load.

Yield: 6–8 SERVINGS

2 tbsp (30 g) coconut oil

1½ cups (210 g) cassava flour

½ cup (60 g) tigernut flour

1 tbsp (14 g) + 1 tsp baking powder

¼ tsp salt

2 tbsp (24 g) coconut sugar

2 eggs

1¼ cups (300 ml) coconut milk

½ cup (120 ml) water

1 cup (148 g) blueberries

Maple syrup, for serving

Turn the Instant Pot to the sauté setting. Add 2 tablespoons (30 g) of coconut oil and allow it to heat while you prepare the pancake. In a medium bowl, whisk together the cassava flour, tigernut flour, baking powder and salt. Set the batter aside.

In a separate bowl, whisk together the coconut sugar, eggs, coconut milk and water. Whisk the dry ingredients into the wet ingredients, making sure everything is well incorporated. Stir in the blueberries.

Very carefully swirl the pot around to make sure the oil is evenly coating the bottom of the pot and then pour the batter into the Instant Pot. Smooth the top with a spoon or spatula and then seal the lid.

Set the Instant Pot to cook for 40 minutes with low pressure on the multigrain setting. When it beeps, quick release the pressure and remove the lid to allow the steam to escape. Allow it to cook for 5 minutes and then gently run an offset spatula or butter knife around the edge of the pancake to make sure it has released. Then, carefully flip the pancake onto a serving plate. Enjoy with some maple syrup.

MINI BLUEBERRY LOAF

Following a low histamine diet is not restrictive whatsoever. This delicious blueberry loaf is just another way to enjoy some sweet bread for breakfast. The quercetin in the blueberries helps keep your histamine bucket low.

Yield: 2 (4-INCH [10-CM]) LOAVES

1½ cups (180 g) tigernut flour

½ cup (70 g) cassava flour

1 tbsp (14 g) + 1 tsp baking powder

½ tsp salt

½ cup (96 g) coconut sugar

2 eggs

½ cup (120 ml) melted grass-fed butter or (110 g) coconut oil, plus more for pans

2 tbsp (30 ml) coconut milk

¾ cups (111 g) fresh or frozen blueberries

¾ cup (180 ml) water

In a medium bowl, whisk together the tigernut flour, cassava flour, baking powder and salt. Set this aside.

In a separate bowl, whisk together the coconut sugar, eggs, grass-fed butter and coconut milk. Whisk the dry ingredients into the wet ingredients, making sure that everything is well incorporated. Stir in the blueberries.

Brush two 4-inch (10-cm) mini loaf pans with melted grass-fed butter or coconut oil and then divide the batter between them. Tent the pans with foil and place them on the trivet in the Instant Pot with ¾ cup (180 ml) of water below. Seal the lid and cook with high pressure for 40 minutes. When finished, quick release the pressure and remove the loaves from the Instant Pot. Immediately remove the foil to allow the steam to escape and let the loaves cool for 10 to 15 minutes before slicing.

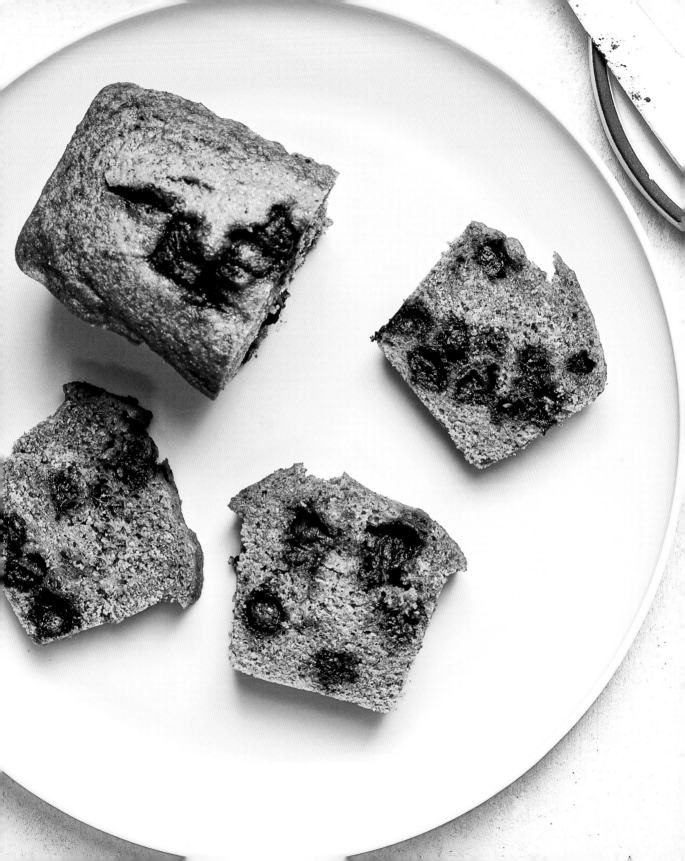

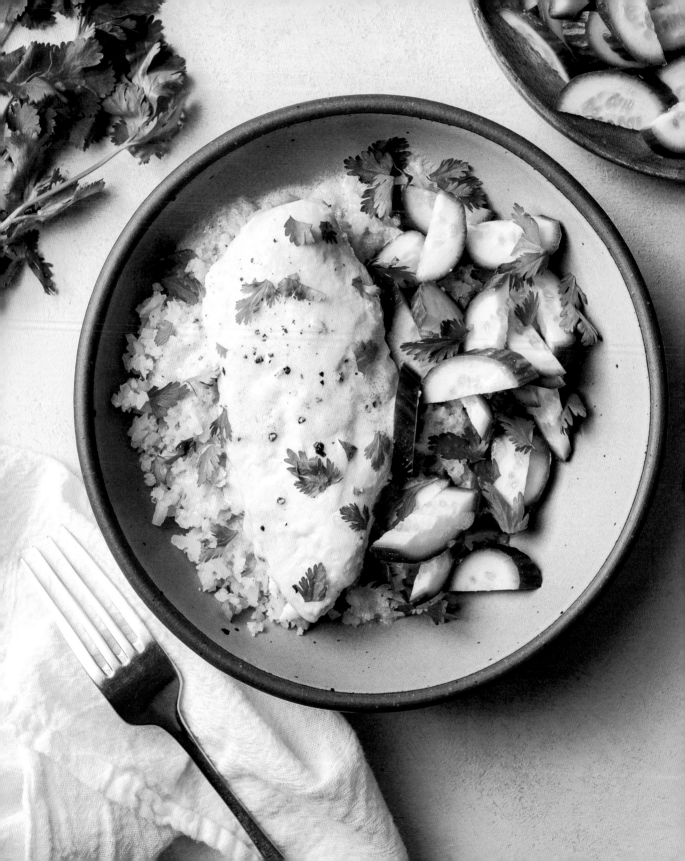

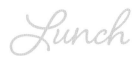

I argue that lunch is just as important as breakfast. A healthy, low histamine lunch will help keep your energy steady in the afternoon. You will have no sugar crashes, afternoon slump or cravings for sugary snacks. A low histamine lunch will also help you stay on track with your low histamine diet for the rest of the day. Whether you are looking for something light or something more elaborate for lunch, you will find some delicious options. The Power Veggie Bowl with Carrot-Ginger Dressing (page 51) and the Broccoli Salad (page 56) are just some of my favorite ones. You will also love the The Perfect Pulled Chicken (page 44) for a protein-rich lunch. Being Instant Pot recipes, they are simple and require no fuss to prepare.

COCONUT–POACHED CHICKEN

This chicken meal is high in proteins and minerals. Thanks to the coconut, it is rich in healthy fats. It is also low in histamine and highly anti-inflammatory. It will soon become one of your favorites.

Yield: 2 SERVINGS

1½ cups (360 ml) coconut milk

½ cup (120 ml) water

1 tsp minced ginger

2 cloves garlic, minced

1 tsp salt

1 bay leaf

2 chicken breasts

Cilantro, to garnish

Whisk the coconut milk, water, ginger, garlic and salt together in the Instant Pot. Add a bay leaf and place the chicken inside.

Seal the lid and cook with high pressure for 10 minutes. Allow the pressure to release naturally for 10 minutes before opening the valve and removing the lid. Remove the bay leaf.

Garnish with the cilantro before serving your chicken on its own, with a salad or with cauliflower rice and cucumbers.

CHICKEN AND CREAMY LEEKS

If you are craving some chicken for lunch, this Chicken and Creamy Leeks recipe is for you. The chicken provides the protein while the leeks offer fiber and minerals, creating a balanced and satisfying meal.

Yield: 2 SERVINGS

1 cup (240 ml) chicken stock

3 leeks, whites cut into ½-inch (1.3-cm) rounds

2 chicken breasts

¼ tsp + a pinch of salt, divided

¼ tsp pepper

2 tbsp (28 g) grass-fed butter

1 clove garlic, minced

1 tsp tapioca flour

1 tbsp (4 g) fresh parsley, for garnish

Pour the chicken stock into the Instant Pot and place the steamer basket inside. Put the leeks in the bottom of the steamer basket and place the chicken breasts side by side on top. Sprinkle the chicken with a pinch of salt and the pepper.

Seal the Instant Pot lid and cook for 10 minutes with high pressure. Quick release the pressure and remove the lid. Carefully remove the steamer basket along with the chicken and leeks from the Instant Pot and switch to sauté.

Add the butter, ¼ teaspoon of salt and the minced garlic to the chicken stock and bring to a boil. Ladle out a small amount of the broth and whisk in the tapioca flour to make a slurry. Pour the slurry back into the pot and whisk well. Allow the sauce to boil for another 5 minutes until it has thickened. Meanwhile, transfer the leeks and chicken to plates.

Pour the warm sauce over the chicken and leeks, and garnish with fresh parsley.

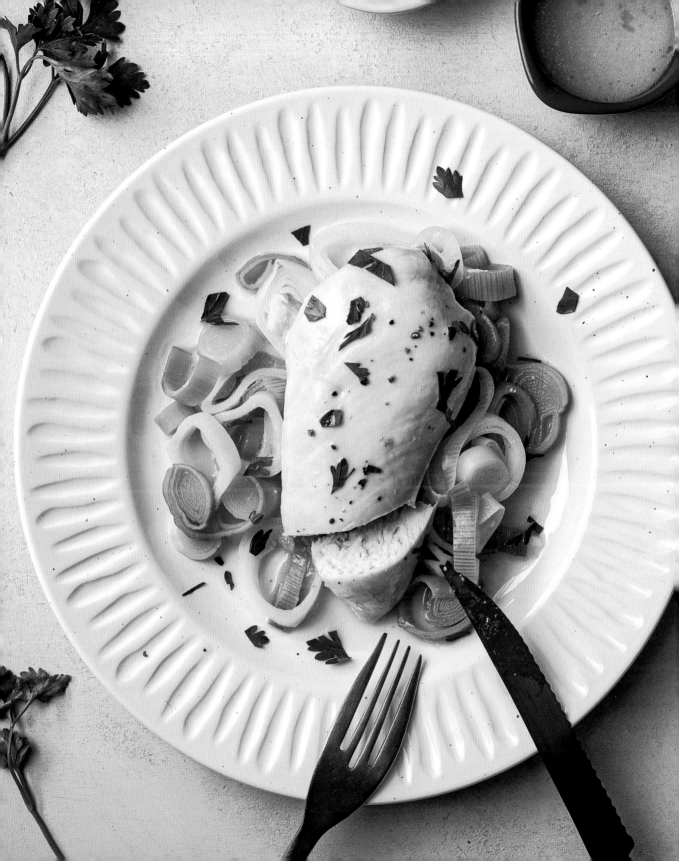

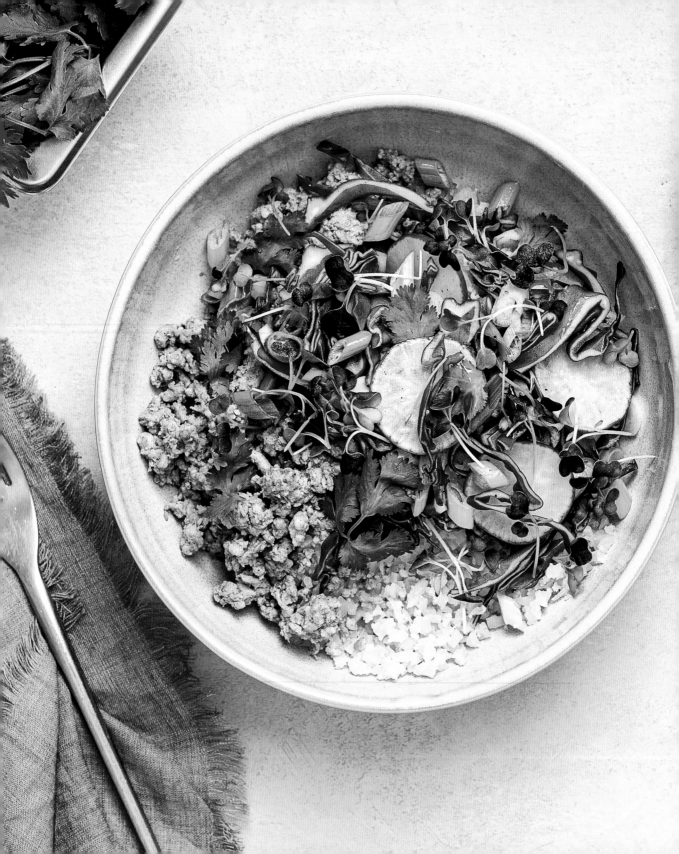

GROUND TURKEY TACO BOWLS

Get ready for Taco Tuesdays, because I have the best recipe for you. It's such a fun and simple recipe and your entire family will love it. Turkey meat is loaded with brain-supporting and energy-boosting B vitamins.

Yield: 4 SERVINGS

4 tbsp (60 ml) olive oil, divided

1 lb (454 g) ground turkey

1 tbsp (8 g) ground cumin

½ tsp + a pinch of salt, divided

½ tsp + a pinch of pepper, divided

¼ cup (60 ml) chicken stock

1 cup (240 ml) water

4 cups (453 g) cauliflower rice

2 radishes, sliced

1 cup (70 g) red cabbage, sliced thin

2 green onions, sliced

½ cup (16 g) microgreens

½ cup (8 g) cilantro leaves

Turn the Instant Pot to the sauté setting. Heat 2 tablespoons (30 ml) of olive oil, then add the ground turkey and cook, stirring often until thoroughly browned, 7 to 10 minutes. Stir in the cumin, ½ teaspoon of salt and ½ teaspoon of pepper. Once the turkey is cooked through, add the chicken stock and cook for an additional 1 to 2 minutes, then transfer the turkey to a bowl and keep covered.

Pour 1 cup (240 ml) of water into the Instant Pot and place the cauliflower rice in a steamer basket inside the pressure cooker. Set the Instant Pot to cook at high pressure for 0 minutes.

While the cauliflower rice is heating, toss together the radishes, cabbage and green onions with the remaining olive oil and a pinch of salt and pepper.

Once the cauliflower rice is finished, divide it among bowls and add the turkey, radish slaw, microgreens and cilantro to each bowl.

THE PERFECT PULLED CHICKEN

Pulled chicken is an easy-to-make and super simple lunch option. It's loaded with protein and low in histamine. It's perfect for energizing you through the rest of the day. Use it in wraps or in salads. There are tons of possibilities!

Yield: 2–3 SERVINGS

1 cup (240 ml) chicken broth

2 chicken breasts

1 tbsp (14 g) grass-fed butter

1 tbsp (4 g) fresh parsley, chopped

Place the broth and chicken breasts in the Instant Pot and seal the lid. Cook with high pressure for 15 minutes.

Quick release the valve and remove the lid. Carefully remove the chicken from the Instant Pot and switch to sauté. Add the butter to the broth and boil until slightly thickened.

Meanwhile, use two forks or your hands to shred the chicken breasts. Drizzle the shredded chicken with some of the buttery broth to keep it moist. Garnish with fresh parsley before serving.

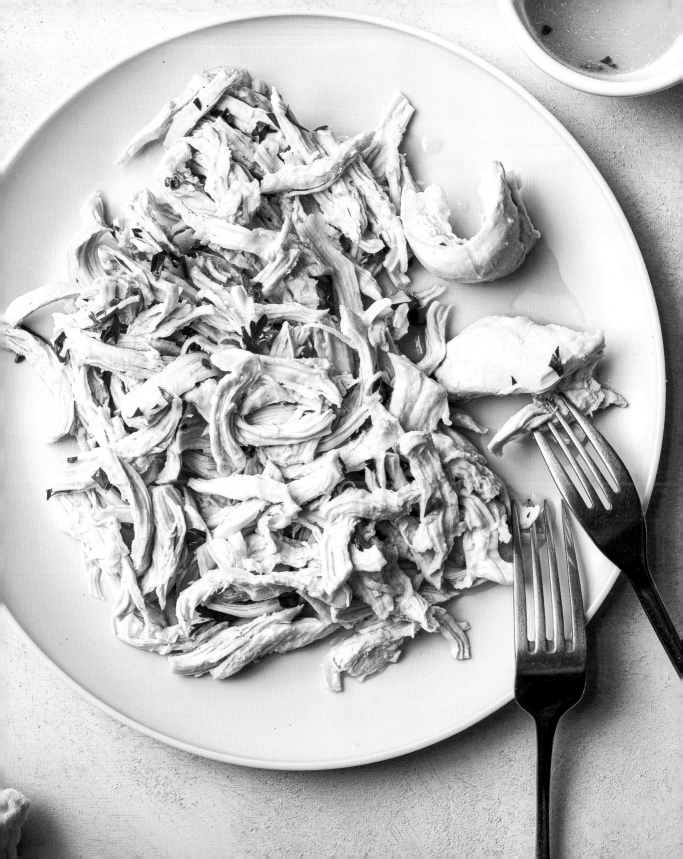

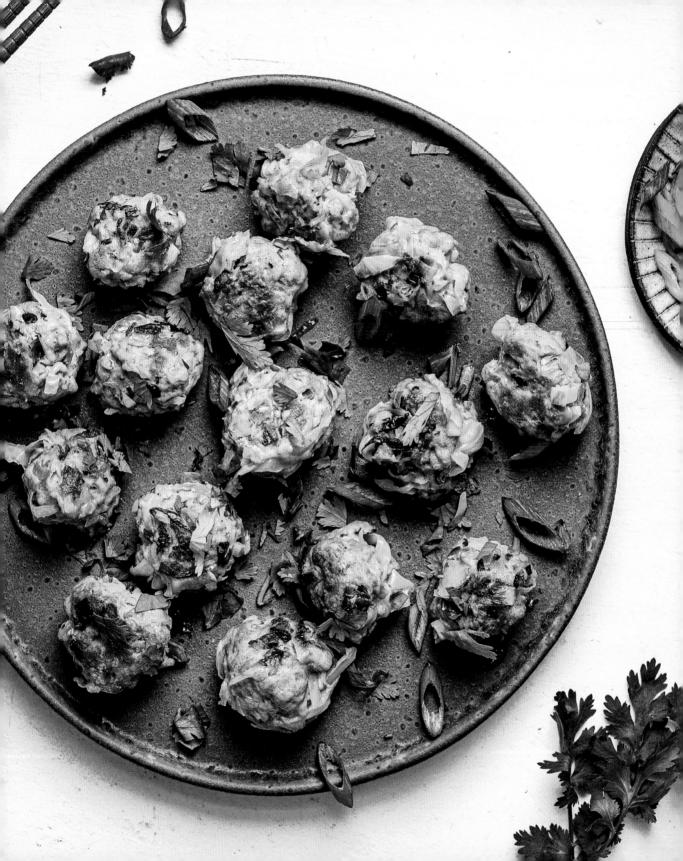

NO-WRAP PORK DUMPLINGS

This is a creative, high-protein lunch option that works for dinner as well. It's full of histamine-lowering quercetin ingredients, such as ginger, cloves, olive oil, pepper, cabbage and cilantro.

Yield: 4 SERVINGS

2 cups (140 g) cabbage, sliced thin

1½ tsp (9 g) salt

1 lb (454 g) ground pork

1 (1-inch [2.5-cm]) piece ginger, minced

3 cloves garlic, minced

½ bunch scallions, sliced

½ tsp pepper

1 cup (240 ml) water

2 tbsp (30 ml) olive oil

¼ cup (4 g) fresh cilantro

Place the sliced cabbage into a medium bowl and sprinkle it with salt. Massage the salt into the cabbage and then allow it to sit for 10 minutes to release moisture.

In a separate bowl, combine the pork, ginger, garlic, scallions and pepper. Squeeze any excess water from the salted cabbage and add to the bowl with the pork. Use your hands to gently squeeze together the contents of the bowl until everything is evenly mixed. Pinch off and separate small pieces of the mixture, about 1½ table-spoons (22 g) in size. Place them into a steamer basket and put them in the Instant Pot with 1 cup (240 ml) of water in the bottom. Make sure that there is space between each dumpling—you may need to work in batches.

Set your Instant Pot to cook with high pressure for 5 minutes. Quick release the pressure, then remove the basket and drain the Instant Pot. Return the pot to the base and turn on the sauté function. Heat the olive oil and then, working in batches, sear the cooked dumplings to create a crisped exterior. They will need only 1 to 2 minutes per side.

Sprinkle the dumplings with cilantro and serve warm.

STUFFED BELL PEPPERS

This is one of my favorite lunch recipes. Peppers are high in histamine-fighting quercetin and rich in antioxidants, vitamins and minerals. The minced beef or lamb offers a healthy dose of protein to keep you strong and help you power through the day.

Yield: 4 BELL PEPPERS

4 bell peppers of any color

2 tbsp (30 ml) olive oil

1 onion, diced

1 lb (454 g) lean ground lamb or beef

1 tsp salt

½ tsp pepper

12 oz (339 g) cauliflower rice

1½ tsp (3 g) dried oregano

1 tbsp (6 g) fresh mint

¼ cup (13 g) fresh dill

¼ cup (60 ml) water

Carefully remove the tops from the bell peppers and pull out any seeds from inside. Keep the tops to place back on the bell peppers before cooking.

Turn the Instant Pot on to sauté. Heat the olive oil and add the diced onion. Cook, stirring occasionally for 3 minutes or until the onion is translucent. Add the ground lamb or beef and stir, breaking the meat apart. Cook for about 10 minutes, stirring often, until the meat has browned all the way through. Add the salt, pepper, cauliflower rice and dried oregano. Cook for another 1 to 2 minutes, then remove from the heat and stir in the fresh mint and dill.

Scoop the lamb mixture into the bell peppers and place the tops back on. Then, place the filled peppers onto the trivet inside the cleaned Instant Pot. Add ¼ cup (60 ml) of water to the pot, seal the lid and cook with high pressure for 7 minutes. Quick release the pressure and serve.

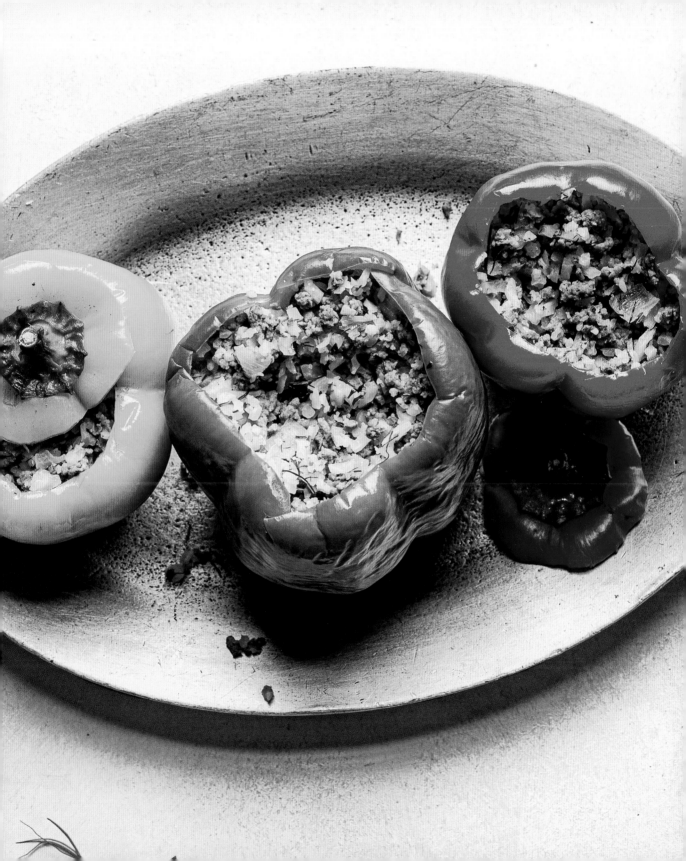

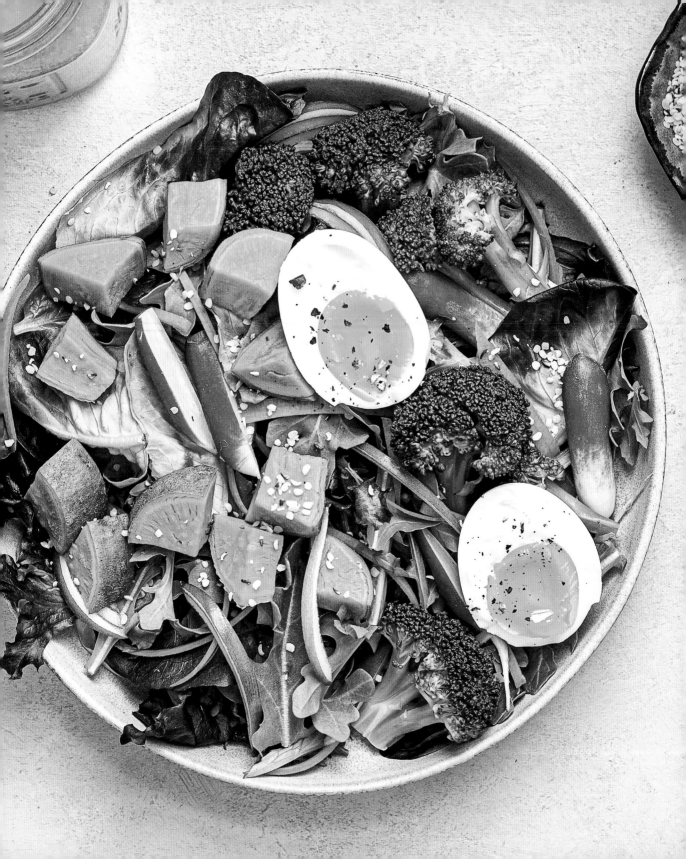

POWER VEGGIE BOWL
WITH CARROT–GINGER DRESSING

You will never have to wonder if you are meeting your daily vegetable needs if you are choosing this power bowl for lunch. It's got fiber, anti-inflammatory benefits, antioxidants and low histamine ingredients—check, check, check and check.

Yield: 2 SERVINGS

FOR THE DRESSING

2 carrots, diced

2 tbsp (30 g) minced ginger

3 tbsp (45 ml) apple cider vinegar (if not tolerated, substitute with distilled white vinegar)

¼ tsp salt

¼ tsp pepper

¼ tsp turmeric

1 clove garlic, minced

⅓ cup (80 ml) olive oil

FOR THE SALAD

2 eggs

1 large sweet potato, diced into 1-inch (2.5-cm) pieces

1 small head broccoli, cut into florets

3 cups (105 g) mixed greens (no spinach)

1 carrot, sliced

¼ red onion, sliced thin

2 tbsp (20 g) hemp seeds

Make the salad dressing by pureeing the carrots, minced ginger, apple cider vinegar, salt, pepper, turmeric, garlic and olive oil in a blender until mostly smooth. Set aside.

Cook the eggs to your liking according to the recipe on page 32, 3 minutes for very soft yolks and 7 minutes for hard-boiled. Remove the eggs from the Instant Pot and run under cold water.

Add the sweet potato and broccoli to a steamer basket and place them in the Instant Pot. Cook with high pressure for 5 minutes and then quick release the pressure and remove.

Divide the mixed greens between the bowls and then top with the broccoli, sweet potato, eggs, carrot, sliced red onion and hemp seeds, then drizzle with the dressing. Extra dressing can be kept in the refrigerator for up to 1 week.

GINGERY CHICKEN SALAD

There is more to a salad than rabbit food. This Gingery Chicken Salad is a complete meal that's loaded with antioxidants. Thanks to the ginger, it fights inflammation and thanks to the chicken, it boosts your protein intake for the day.

Yield: 2 SERVINGS

FOR THE LOW HISTAMINE MAYONNAISE (MAKES 1 CUP [240 ML])

1 large egg (if sensitive to egg whites, replace with 2 egg yolks)

1½ tbsp (20 g) mustard made with distilled white vinegar (such as Annie's® brand)

1 cup (240 ml) extra-light tasting olive oil

½ tsp sea salt

FOR THE CHICKEN SALAD

2 chicken breasts

1 cup (240 ml) water

¼ cup (60 ml) Low Histamine Mayonnaise

½ tsp salt

¼ tsp pepper

2 tsp (2 g) ground ginger

⅓ cup (50 g) seedless red grapes, sliced or quartered

2 ribs celery, thinly sliced

4 scallions, sliced

2 tbsp (4 g) fresh tarragon, chopped

First, make the mayonnaise by placing the egg, mustard, olive oil and salt in a mason jar and then stick in an emulsion blender all the way to the bottom. Once the bottom portion is emulsified, slowly bring the blender up and blend until the next portion is emulsified, going up and down as necessary to create a homogenous mixture. Repeat this process until the mixture is creamy throughout, for about 1 to 2 minutes. Set aside ¼ of the mayonnaise for the salad and store the rest in the refrigerator.

Place the chicken breasts on the trivet in the Instant Pot with the water in the bottom. Seal the lid and cook on the high pressure setting for 10 minutes. Quick release the pressure and then remove the chicken breasts from the Instant Pot and allow to cool.

Meanwhile, in a large bowl, whisk together the mayonnaise, salt, pepper and ginger. When the chicken is cool, dice into ½-inch (1.3-cm) cubes and add them to the bowl with the mayonnaise, along with the grapes, celery, scallions and tarragon. Stir and then taste and adjust the seasoning as necessary.

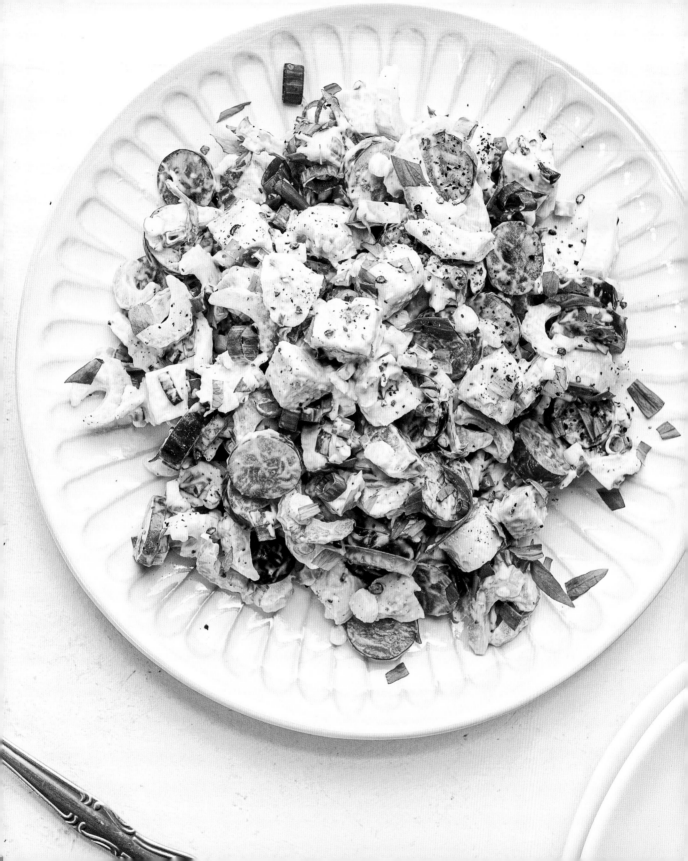

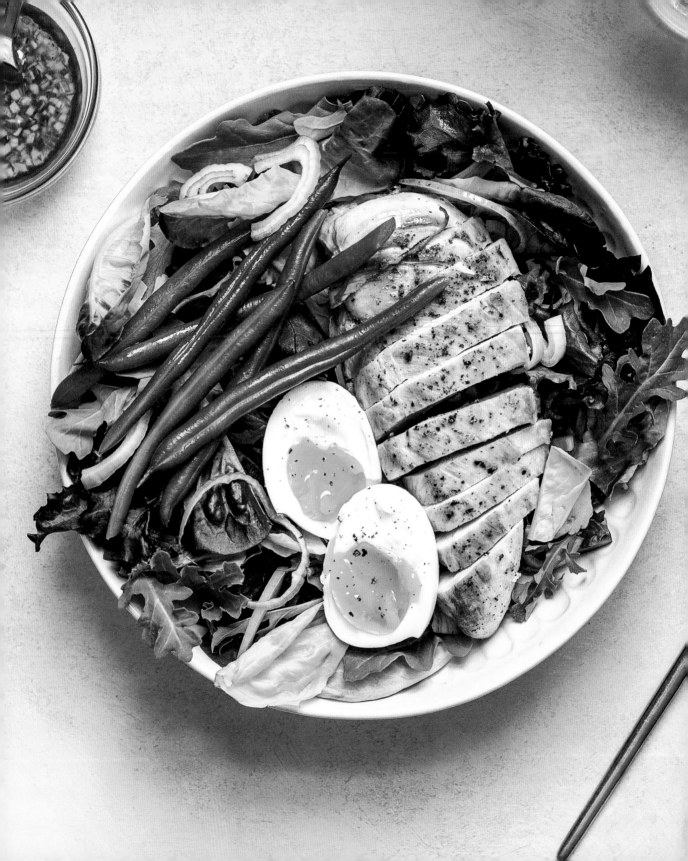

ALMOST NIÇOISE SALAD

This is a gourmet salad, yet it's so easy to make at home. If you are looking for a protein fix within a light meal, this salad offers a great option with two protein sources, chicken and eggs. It also adds a good amount of veggies to your daily micronutrient bucket.

Yield: 2 SERVINGS

FOR THE HONEY-SHALLOT VINAIGRETTE

1 tbsp (15 ml) honey

1 tbsp (10 g) minced shallot

2 tsp (10 ml) apple cider vinegar

Pinch of salt and pepper

⅓ cup (80 ml) olive oil

FOR THE SALAD

2 eggs

2 tbsp (30 ml) olive oil

Pinch of salt

Pinch of pepper

2 chicken breasts

½ cup (55 g) green beans

1 cup (240 ml) water

3 cups (105 g) mixed salad greens (no spinach)

¼ shallot, sliced

Make the vinaigrette by mixing together the honey, minced shallot, apple cider vinegar, salt and pepper in a small bowl. Whisk everything together while slowly streaming in the olive oil. Set the vinaigrette aside while you prepare the salad.

Cook the eggs according to the recipe on page 32, 3 minutes for very soft yolks and 7 minutes for hard-boiled eggs. Once they are done cooking, run the eggs under cold water and then remove the shells and slice in half.

Use the sauté setting to sear the chicken breasts. Heat the olive oil in the pot and sprinkle a pinch of salt and pepper onto the chicken breasts. Sear on both sides until browned, about 5 minutes for each side. Use tongs to remove the breasts from the Instant Pot and transfer them to a steamer basket along with the green beans. Pour the water into the pot and then put the steamer basket inside and cook with high pressure for 7 minutes.

Quick release the pressure and then transfer the chicken to a cutting board and slice it.

Divide the salad greens between two bowls and top with the chicken, green beans, eggs, sliced shallot and vinaigrette.

BROCCOLI SALAD

Here is more proof that salads don't have to be boring. Thanks to the broccoli, this salad is a high-quercetin and low histamine lunch option. The almonds provide healthy fats, fiber, magnesium, vitamin E and some crunch.

Yield: 2-4 SERVINGS

1 cup (240 ml) water

1 large head broccoli, cut into florets

⅓ cup (80 ml) Low Histamine Mayonnaise (page 52)

½ tsp salt

¼ tsp pepper

1 tsp apple cider vinegar (optional)

1 carrot, cut into matchsticks

½ red onion, sliced thin

1 cup (70 g) purple cabbage, sliced thin

¼ cup (27 g) slivered almonds, toasted (omit if not tolerated)

Place the steamer basket into the Instant Pot with the water. Put the broccoli in the basket and seal the lid. Cook with high pressure for 1 minute, quick release the pressure and then remove the broccoli and run it under cool water to stop the cooking process. Allow it to drain while you prepare the remaining ingredients.

In a large bowl, whisk together the mayonnaise, salt, pepper and apple cider vinegar, if using. Add the broccoli, carrot, onion and cabbage to the bowl and toss to evenly coat with dressing. Add 1 to 2 tablespoons (15 to 30 ml) more of the mayonnaise, if desired. Top with the toasted almond slices.

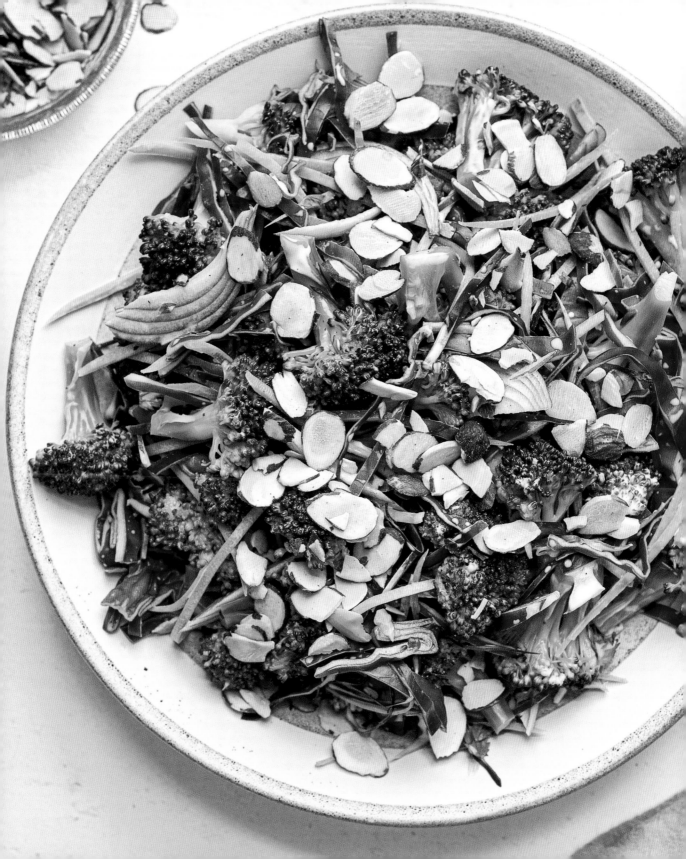

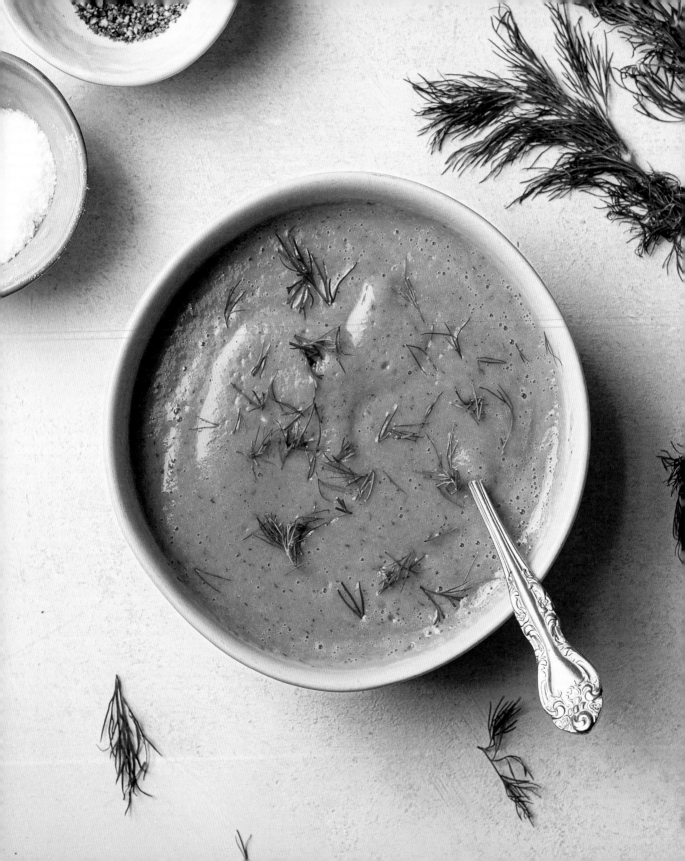

ASPARAGUS AND DILL SOUP

Asparagus is high in fiber and low in histamine. It is highly anti-inflammatory, just like dill. Enjoying this delicious Asparagus and Dill Soup is easy on your digestion and good for your health.

Yield: 2-3 SERVINGS

1 large bunch asparagus

½ head cauliflower, quartered

1 onion, quartered

3 cups (720 ml) chicken or vegetable stock

2 cloves garlic

½ tsp salt

¼ tsp pepper

2 tbsp (7 g) fresh dill, plus more for garnish

1 tsp apple cider vinegar (omit if not tolerated)

Grass-fed butter, for garnish

Trim the woody bottoms off of the asparagus, ½ to 1 inch (1.3 to 2.5 cm), and place the asparagus in the Instant Pot with the cauliflower, onion, chicken stock, garlic, salt and pepper.

Seal the lid and cook with high pressure for 8 minutes. Allow the pressure to release naturally for 10 to 15 minutes before opening the Instant Pot. Transfer the contents to a blender and add the dill and apple cider vinegar, if using. Blend the ingredients on high until the soup is smooth—you might still see specks of dill, but that's okay.

Taste and adjust the seasoning if necessary. Garnish with a small pat of butter and dill.

CREAMY CAULIFLOWER SOUP

One of the main concerns with creamy soups is their dairy content. You don't have to worry about this with this dairy-free recipe. Thanks to the addition of cauliflower, this soup is loaded with histamine-reducing quercetin. It's also creamy and satisfying without causing you to worry about inflammation from dairy products.

Yield: 3-4 SERVINGS

1 medium cauliflower, roughly chopped

1 leek or 2 shallots, roughly chopped

1 clove garlic

½ tsp salt

2 tbsp (28 g) grass-fed butter

1 sprig rosemary, left whole

2 cups (480 ml) vegetable broth

1 tbsp (5 g) nutritional yeast

Salt and pepper, to taste

Olive oil, for serving

Place the cauliflower, leek or shallots, garlic, salt, butter, rosemary sprig and vegetable broth into the Instant Pot and seal the lid. Cook with high pressure for 10 minutes and then slow release the pressure for 10 minutes before opening.

Remove the rosemary stalk and transfer the remaining ingredients along with the nutritional yeast to a blender. Blend everything until smooth. Taste and adjust the seasoning with salt and pepper. Serve with a drizzle of olive oil.

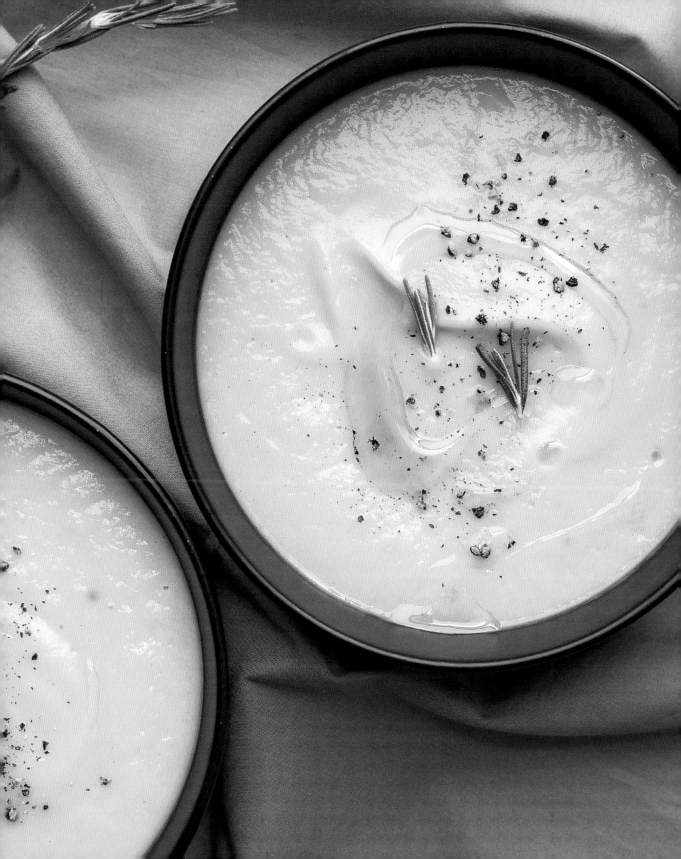

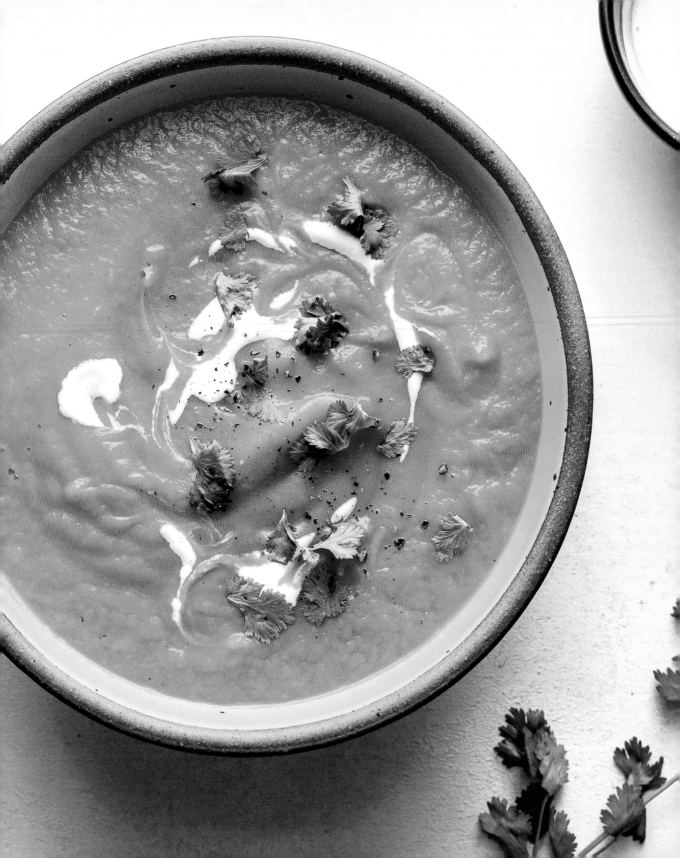

THAI–STYLE CARROT SOUP

This Asian-inspired soup is another nourishing liquid lunch that's smooth on your digestion. Coconut milk offers anti-inflammatory benefits and makes it a filling midday meal. Lemongrass helps to fight bacteria, yeast infections and pain. It also provides a unique and delicious flavor.

Yield: 2-3 SERVINGS

2 lb (908 g) carrots, peeled and cut into 1-inch (2.5-cm) sections

1-inch (2.5-cm) piece lemongrass

½-inch (1.3-cm) piece ginger, diced

1 onion, quartered

1 cup (240 ml) vegetable stock

1 cup (240 ml) coconut milk, plus 2 tbsp (30 ml) for garnish

½ tsp salt, plus more to taste

¼ tsp pepper, plus more to taste

¼ tsp coriander seeds (optional)

1 bay leaf

1 tbsp (1 g) cilantro, for garnish

Place the carrots, lemongrass, ginger, onion, vegetable stock, coconut milk, salt, pepper, coriander seeds (if using) and bay leaf into the Instant Pot. Close the lid and cook with high pressure for 8 minutes. Slowly release the steam for 10 minutes, then remove the bay leaf and transfer all the remaining ingredients to a blender.

Blend the soup until smooth. Taste and adjust the seasoning with salt and pepper. Garnish with coconut milk and cilantro.

PARSNIP SOUP

I cannot recommend this soup for lunch enough. It's loaded with nutrients and easy on your digestion. Parsnip is high in fiber, potassium, folate and vitamin C. It's also anti-inflammatory, antifungal and low histamine.

Yield: 3 SERVINGS

6 large parsnips

3 carrots

1 onion

4 cups (960 ml) chicken or vegetable stock

½ tsp salt, plus more to taste

¼ tsp pepper, plus more to taste

2–3 tbsp (30–45 ml) olive oil, for drizzling

Fresh parsley and scallions, for garnish

Chop the parsnips, carrots and onion into large, evenly sized pieces and place them in the Instant Pot along with the chicken stock, salt and pepper. Seal the lid and cook with high pressure for 7 minutes. Allow the pressure to release naturally for 10 minutes before releasing the valve and opening the lid.

Transfer all of the contents to a blender, working in batches if necessary, and blend on high until smooth. Taste the soup and adjust the salt and pepper as desired. Serve with a drizzle of olive oil and fresh parsley and scallions.

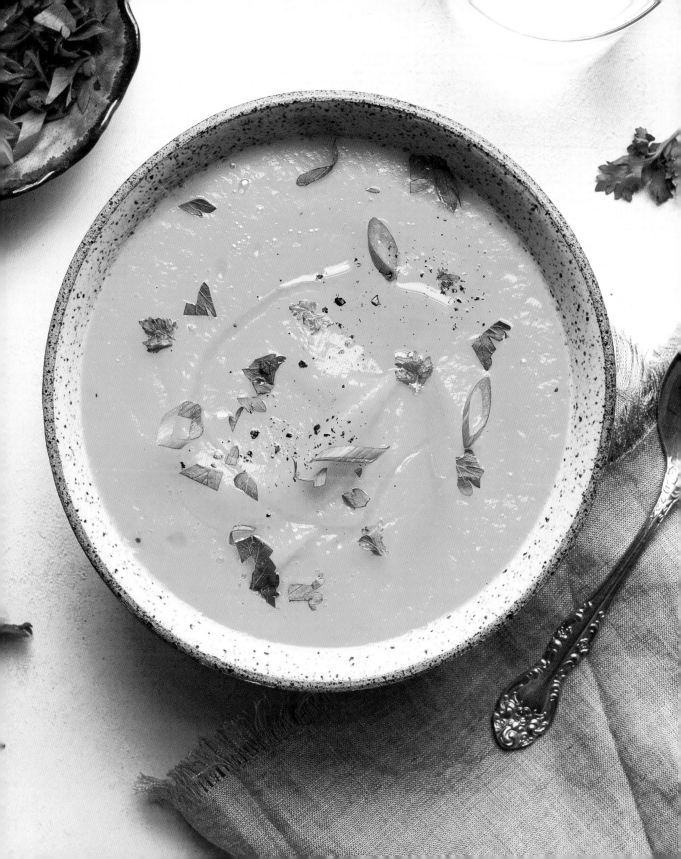

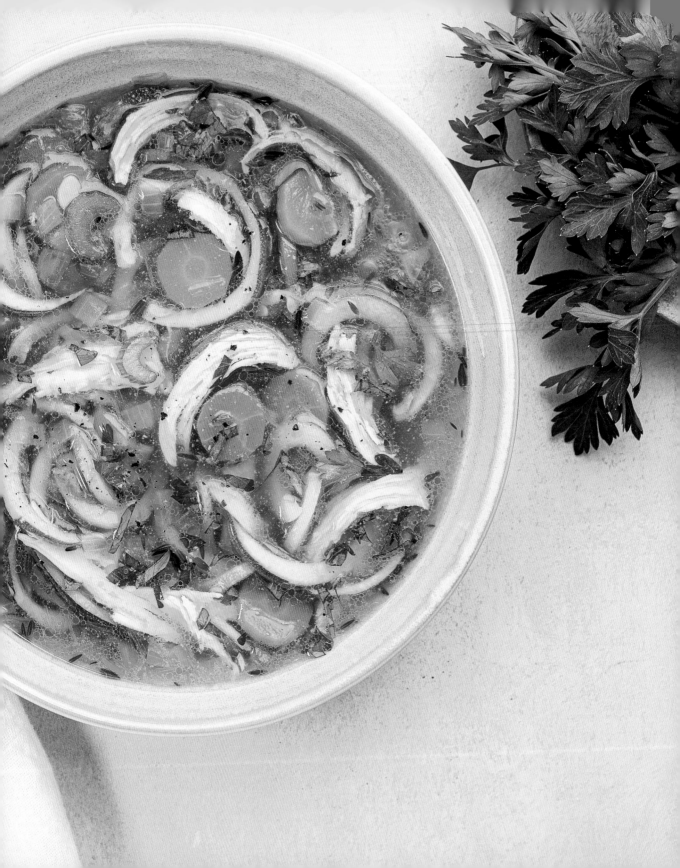

CHICKEN ZOODLE SOUP

Who needs noodles when you have zoodles? It's more fun to say and even more nourishing to eat. This soup is easy on your digestion and low in histamine. You can't ask for more.

Yield: 3-4 SERVINGS

2 tbsp (30 ml) olive oil

3 ribs celery, sliced

3 carrots, sliced into rounds

1 onion, diced

Pinch of salt

Pinch of pepper

2 cloves garlic, minced

4 cups (960 ml) chicken stock

2 chicken breasts

2-3 sprigs fresh thyme

½ lb (227 g) zoodles, from 2 large zucchini

2 tbsp (8 g) fresh parsley, chopped

Turn on the sauté function and allow the Instant Pot to heat for 1 to 2 minutes before pouring the olive oil into the pot.

Sauté the celery, carrots and onion with a pinch of salt and pepper for 3 to 5 minutes or until just tender. Add the garlic and cook for another minute.

Turn off the Instant Pot and add the chicken stock, chicken breasts and thyme.

Seal the lid and cook with high pressure for 10 minutes. Slow release the pressure for 10 minutes, then open the quick release valve and remove the lid.

Transfer the chicken breast to a cutting board to shred and put the zucchini noodles into the hot broth. Turn on the sauté function to bring the soup back to a boil and cook the zucchini noodles for 3 to 5 minutes while you shred the chicken breast.

Place the shredded chicken back into the soup and transfer to bowls for serving. Garnish with fresh parsley.

GREEN MINESTRONE

Who doesn't love a good minestrone soup? It's hearty and filling but also smooth on your digestion. This green minestrone soup is loaded with low histamine vegetables and nourishes your body with vitamins, minerals, antioxidants and fiber.

Yield: 2–3 SERVINGS

1 zucchini, halved lengthwise and sliced

2 celery ribs, sliced

1 cup (110 g) green beans

1 onion, sliced

4 cloves garlic, minced

3 cups (720 ml) chicken stock

½ tsp salt

½ tsp pepper

½ cup (12 g) fresh basil, for serving

Add the zucchini, celery, green beans, onion, garlic, chicken stock, salt and pepper to the Instant Pot, and seal the lid. Cook with high pressure for 5 minutes.

Allow the pressure to release naturally for 10 minutes and then remove the lid. Serve with fresh basil leaves.

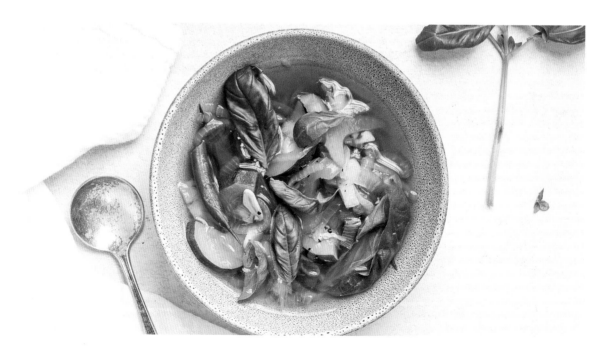

SWEET POTATO CHOWDER

If you are looking for something warm and satisfying, look no further. This sweet potato chowder is absolutely delicious. Sweet potatoes are low in histamine and, because this dish is a soup, it is also easy on your digestion.

Yield: 2–3 SERVINGS

2 sweet potatoes, peeled and diced into ½-inch (1.3-cm) pieces

1 onion, diced

2 celery ribs, diced

1 clove garlic, minced

2 cups (480 ml) chicken or vegetable stock

1 cup (240 ml) coconut milk

½ tsp salt, plus more to taste

Chives, to garnish

Place the sweet potatoes, onion, celery, garlic, chicken stock, coconut milk and salt into the Instant Pot and seal the lid. Cook with high pressure for 6 minutes. Quick release the pressure, and then transfer half of the chowder to a blender and blend until smooth. Add it back to the Instant Pot and stir well. Taste and adjust the salt as necessary. Garnish with fresh chives before serving.

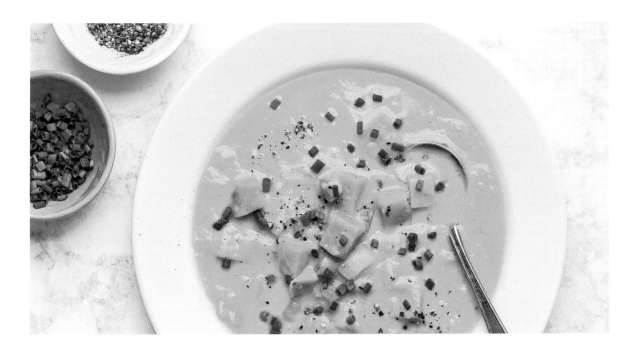

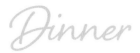

Dinner

You've made it. Dinner is the last meal of your day, except for dessert, of course! A nourishing, low histamine dinner is the perfect way to end your day. A hearty, healthy and low histamine dinner will help you feel satisfied for the rest of the night and help you sleep soundly without hunger pangs or cravings. Remember, you can always pair your dinner with any of my low histamine side options for a more elaborate, delicious meal. There are so many options. For a family meal, try my Garlic Butter Chicken (below). For an international-inspired meal, I recommend my Tortilla-less Green Chicken Enchiladas (page 74). If you are feeling under the weather or need a boost of immune-supporting nutrients, try my Healing Chicken Soup with Ginger and Turmeric (page 98).

GARLIC BUTTER CHICKEN

This delicious, healthy meal is rich in protein and healthy fat thanks to the chicken and butter. The thyme, garlic and parsley provide antihistamine, anti-inflammatory and antioxidant benefits.

Yield: 4 SERVINGS

1 cup (240 ml) water

1 lb (454 g) chicken tenders or breasts, cubed

3 tbsp (42 g) grass-fed butter

3 cloves garlic, minced

5 sprigs fresh thyme

1 tbsp (2 g) fresh parsley, chopped

½ tsp salt

¼ tsp pepper

Pour the water into the Instant Pot and place the steamer basket inside. Put the cubed chicken into the basket and seal the Instant Pot lid. Set to cook with high pressure for 10 minutes. Once finished, quick release the pressure, remove the basket with the chicken and drain the water from the Instant Pot.

Return the pot to the base and turn on the sauté function. Add the butter, garlic, thyme sprigs, parsley, salt and pepper to the Instant Pot, and allow everything to heat until the butter is melted. Add the chicken to the pot and cook, stirring occasionally, until the chicken and garlic begin to crisp and brown.

Remove from the Instant Pot and serve.

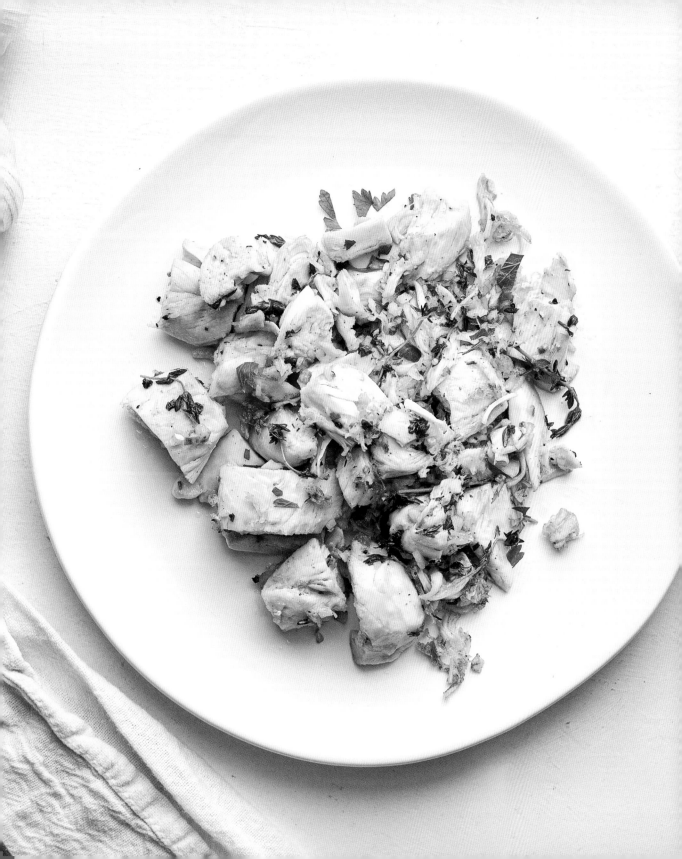

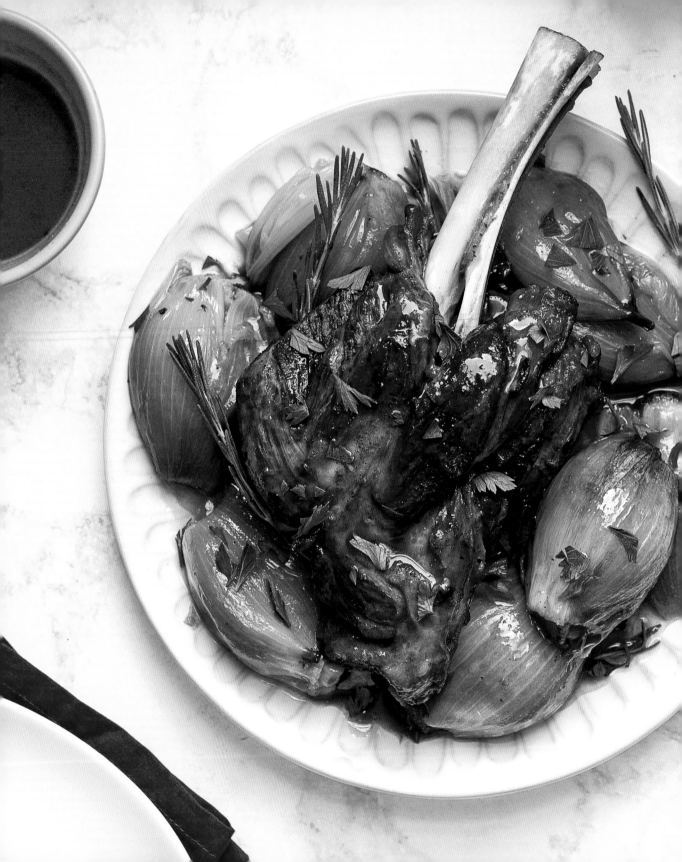

LAMB SHANK WITH SHALLOTS

This meal is an antihistamine powerhouse. The salt, pepper, cumin, rosemary and bay leaf all possess antihistamine and anti-inflammatory benefits. Olive oil is a great source of healthy fats and lamb is a nourishing clean protein.

Yield: 3–4 SERVINGS

1 tsp salt

½ tsp pepper

1 tsp cumin

2–3 lb (908 g–1.4 kg) lamb shank or leg of lamb

2 tbsp (30 ml) olive oil

8–10 shallots, peeled and whole

1 cup (240 ml) vegetable or beef broth

2 sprigs rosemary

1 bay leaf

1 tbsp (10 g) chopped parsley, for garnish

In a small bowl, mix the salt, pepper and cumin. Pat the lamb dry and rub the salt mixture on all sides. Heat the olive oil in the Instant Pot on the sauté setting and sear the lamb on all sides, around 5 minutes per side. If the lamb doesn't sit flat in the Instant Pot, this step can be done in a cast-iron skillet.

Add the shallots, vegetable broth, rosemary sprigs and bay leaf to the Instant Pot along with the seared lamb and seal the lid. Set to cook with high pressure for 30 minutes and then quick release the pressure, carefully remove the lamb and shallots and set aside. Discard the bay leaf. Turn the sauté setting back on and allow the broth to reduce slightly while the lamb rests. Spoon the broth over the lamb and shallots and garnish with parsley before serving.

TORTILLA–LESS GREEN CHICKEN ENCHILADAS

Enchiladas are delicious. The problem is that conventional recipes use tortillas made with inflammatory, gluten-filled flour or corn. To prevent inflammation and histamine intolerance, I recommend that you try this Tortilla-less Green Chicken Enchiladas recipe.

Yield: 3 SERVINGS

2 tbsp (30 ml) olive oil

1 zucchini, cut in half lengthwise and sliced

1 onion, sliced

2 poblano peppers, sliced

2 cloves garlic, minced

¾ cup (180 ml) chicken stock

1 tsp cumin

½ tsp salt, plus more to taste

¼ tsp pepper, plus more to taste

2 chicken breasts

1 cup (16 g) cilantro leaves, plus more for garnish

Turn the Instant Pot onto the sauté setting and heat the olive oil. Cook the zucchini, onion and poblano peppers until slightly softened, about 5 minutes.

Add the garlic, chicken stock, cumin, salt, pepper and chicken breasts. Seal the lid and cook with high pressure for 10 minutes. Quick release the pressure and remove the chicken to a cutting board.

Carefully transfer half of the vegetables and stock to a blender or food processor. Add 1 cup (16 g) of cilantro and puree until mostly smooth. Taste and adjust the salt and pepper as necessary.

Shred the chicken and place in a medium bowl with the remaining vegetables. Toss with the green cilantro sauce and garnish with cilantro.

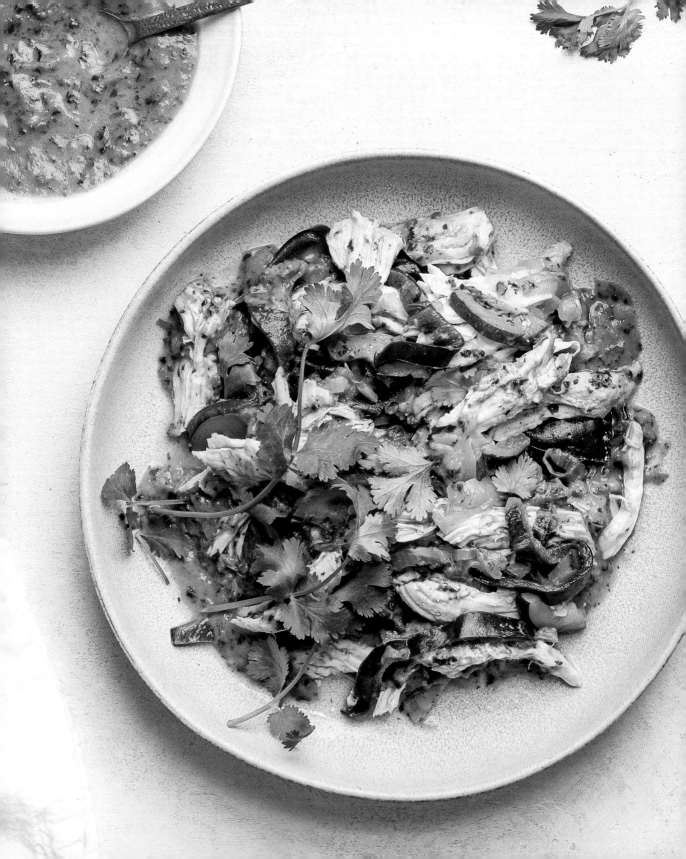

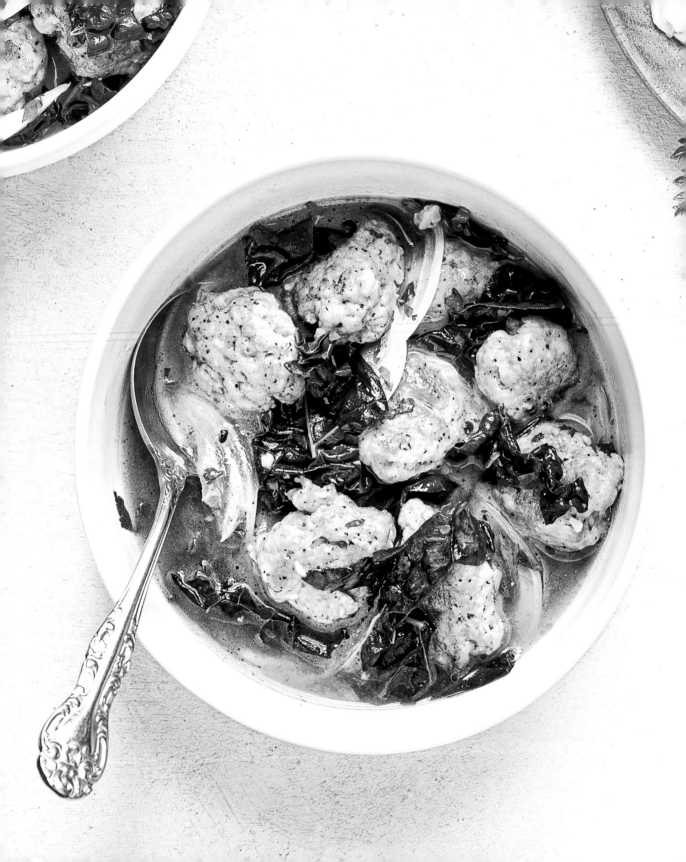

SAUSAGE AND KALE STEW

This recipe is perfect for colder days or if you are craving some comfort food. Dried sausage tends to contain more histamine, so I am using sweet Italian sausage instead, which is not triggering for most. The kale, onion, garlic and salt in this recipe all offer histamine-lowering effects while helping you meet your vegetable needs for the day.

Yield: 4 SERVINGS

1 lb (454 g) sweet Italian sausage, no casing

2 tbsp (30 ml) olive oil

2 bunches kale or other dark leafy green such as Swiss chard, roughly chopped

2 cloves garlic, minced

1½ cups (360 ml) vegetable stock

Pinch of salt

Pinch of pepper

2 tbsp (28 g) grass-fed butter

1 tsp tapioca flour

½ small onion, sliced paper thin

2 tbsp (8 g) fresh parsley, to garnish

Break the sausage meat into 1-inch (2.5-cm) pieces. Turn the Instant Pot to the sauté setting and heat the olive oil. Sear the sausage pieces for 2 to 3 minutes on each side, until they are browned.

Once the sausage is cooked, add the kale, garlic and vegetable stock with a pinch of salt and pepper, and seal the lid. Cook with high pressure for 5 minutes. Quick release the pressure and then use tongs to remove the sausage and kale, and divide among bowls for serving. Turn the Instant Pot on the sauté setting and add the butter. Remove ¼ cup (60 ml) of broth to a bowl and whisk in the tapioca flour. Then, return the slurry to the Instant Pot, pouring through a strainer if there are lumps. Continue to cook the broth for a few more minutes until slightly thickened, and then ladle into bowls with the sausage and kale. Place a few slices of raw onion into each bowl and garnish with fresh parsley.

EASY BEEF STEW WITH CARROT AND SWEET POTATO

This is the simplest beef stew recipe you will find. Beef is extremely rich in minerals and helps to lower the risk of iron deficient anemia. Carrots and sweet potatoes provide some sweetness without throwing off your blood sugar. They are anti-inflammatory and gut-supporting thanks to all the fiber and micronutrients.

Yield: 4 SERVINGS

2 tbsp (30 ml) olive oil

1½ lb (681 g) beef stewing meat, cut into cubes

½ tsp + a pinch of salt, divided

½ tsp + a pinch of pepper, divided

4 carrots

2 medium sweet potatoes,

1 onion, diced

½ cup (66 g) diced raw yuca cassava

2 cups (480 ml) beef stock

3–4 sprigs fresh thyme and rosemary, plus more for garnish

Turn the Instant Pot on to the sauté setting and add the olive oil to the pot. Season the beef with a pinch of salt and pepper and sear until browned on all sides, 3 to 5 minutes per side. You'll need to work in batches or you can use a large cast-iron skillet to sear the meat.

While the meat is cooking, cut the carrots and the sweet potatoes into large, evenly sized pieces. You'll want to make sure the pieces are not too small, as they'll fall apart during the longer cooking time. Aim for about 2-inch (5-cm) pieces.

Return the cooked meat to the Instant Pot and add the carrots, sweet potatoes, onion, yuca cassava, beef stock and sprigs of rosemary and thyme. Seal the lid and set the Instant Pot to cook with high pressure for 25 minutes.

Slow release the pressure, and then serve with fresh thyme and rosemary.

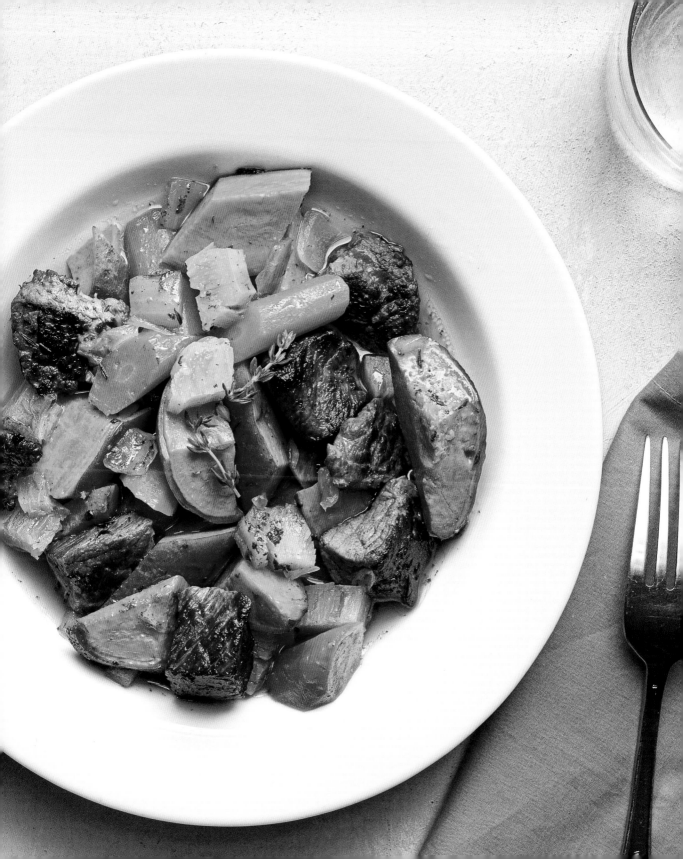

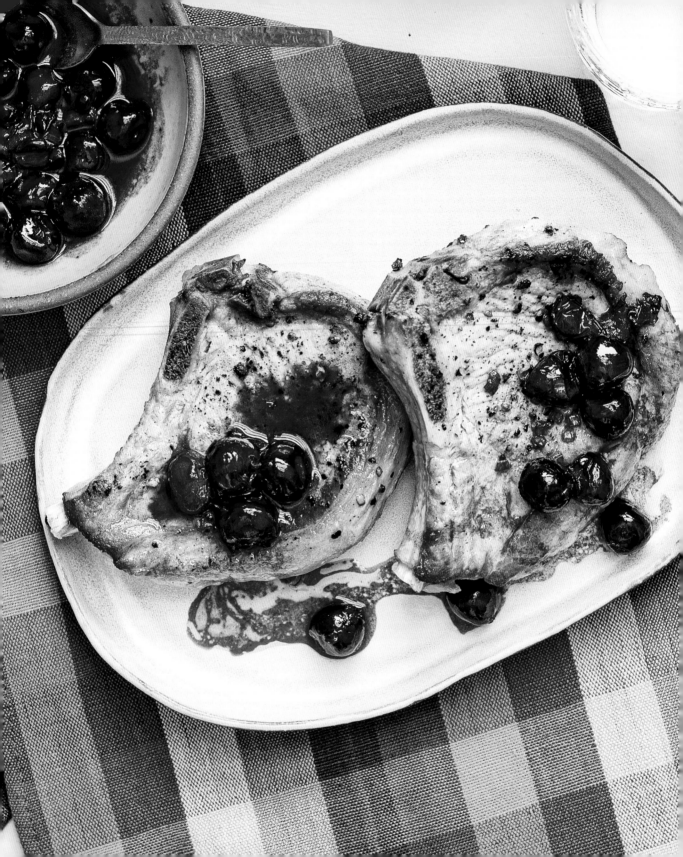

PORK CHOPS WITH CHERRY SAUCE

I love making this tasty anti-inflammatory recipe for dinner. Rosemary and cherries are both rich in quercetin, which is known for its histamine-fighting properties. Pork is incredibly rich in minerals, especially thiamine, selenium, phosphorus, zinc and iron.

Yield: 2 SERVINGS

2 pork chops, approximately 1½ inches (4 cm) thick

Pinch of salt

Pinch of pepper

2 tbsp (30 ml) olive oil

1 cup (240 ml) + 2 tbsp (30 ml) water, divided

¾ cup (116 g) frozen cherries

1 tbsp (10 g) minced shallot

2 tbsp (28 g) grass-fed butter

Season the pork chops with a pinch of salt and pepper on each side.

Turn on the Instant Pot to the sauté setting and heat the olive oil. Sear the pork chops until golden brown on each side, 5 to 7 minutes per side.

Remove the pork chops and add 1 cup (240 ml) of water to the Instant Pot. Place the trivet inside and then place the pork chops on the trivet. Cook with high pressure for 14 minutes and then quick release the pressure and remove the pork.

Drain the water from the Instant Pot and return to the base. Switch back to the sauté setting. Put the cherries, shallot, butter and 2 tablespoons (30 ml) of water in the Instant Pot. Sauté for 5 to 6 minutes, until the cherries have released some liquid and made a sauce.

Drizzle the warm cherry sauce over the pork chops and serve.

WHOLE CHICKEN WITH PEARL ONIONS

This chicken recipe is bringing you the most antihistamine and anti-inflammatory powers thanks to the abundance of herbs like oregano, rosemary, pepper, garlic powder and onion powder. The chicken and butter provide plenty of clean protein and healthy fats for an evening meal.

Yield: 4 SERVINGS

1 tsp salt

1 tsp garlic powder

1 tsp onion powder

1 tsp oregano

1 tsp dried thyme

½ tsp pepper

1 whole chicken

1 cup (240 ml) water

2 cups (258 g) pearl onions

½ cup (120 ml) chicken stock

2 tbsp (28 g) grass-fed butter

2–3 sprigs rosemary

In a small bowl, mix together the salt, garlic powder, onion powder, oregano, thyme and pepper. Rub the seasoning all over the chicken and then place the chicken on the trivet in the Instant Pot with the water below. Seal the lid and cook with high pressure for 6 minutes per pound (454 g) of chicken.

Slow release the pressure for 10 minutes and then transfer the chicken to a serving plate—make sure to drain any water that has collected in the cavity first. Empty the Instant Pot and return to the base.

Add the onions and the chicken stock to the Instant Pot along with the butter and rosemary. Seal the lid and cook with high pressure for 5 minutes and then quick release the pressure and remove the lid. Switch to the sauté setting and allow the broth to come to a boil and simmer until slightly thickened, about 5 minutes. Serve alongside the chicken.

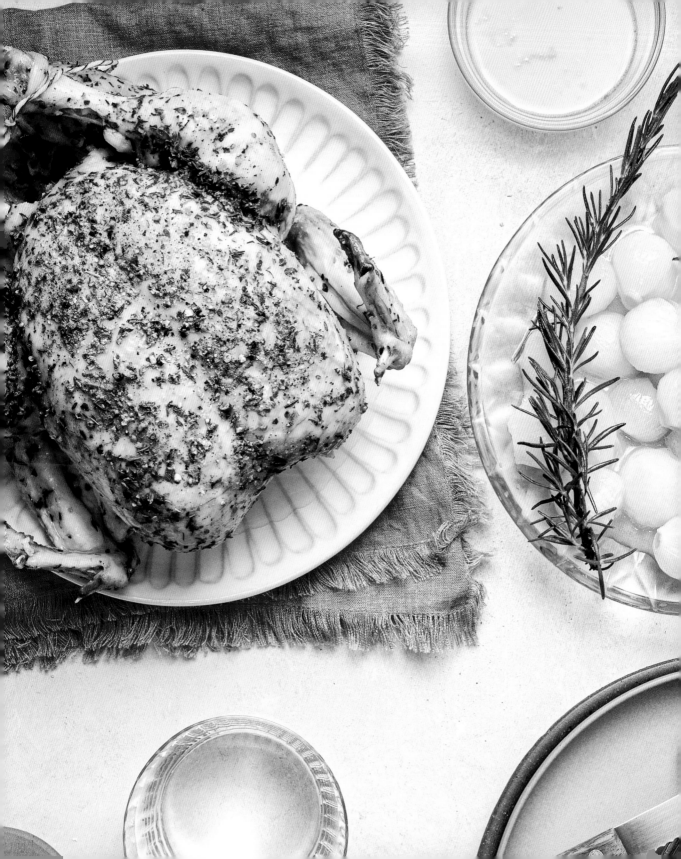

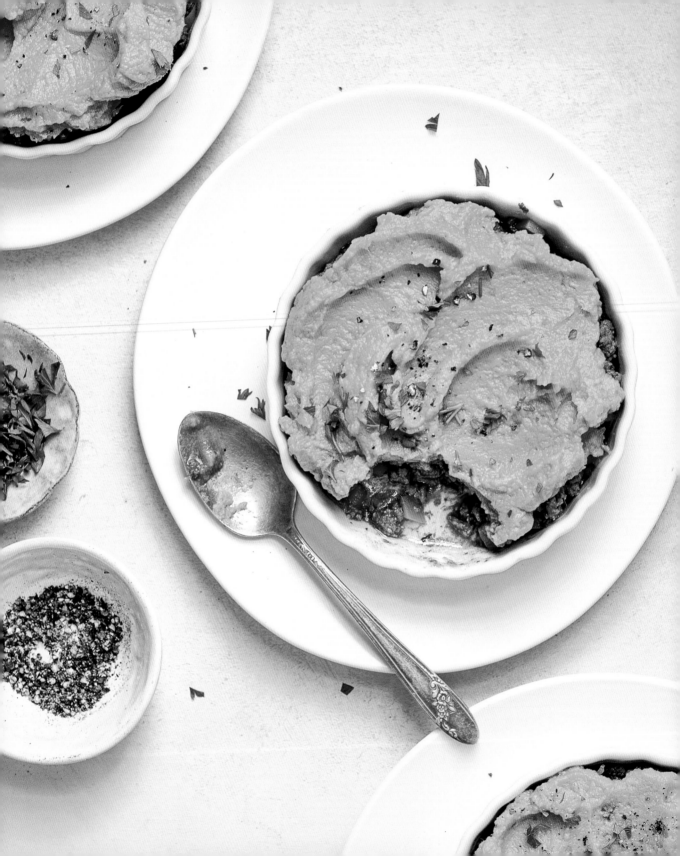

SWEET POTATO SHEPHERD'S PIE

This is comfort food at its finest, except that this meal doesn't raise your histamine levels or interfere with your digestion. It offers ground beef for clean protein, sweet potatoes and carrots for histamine-friendly healthy carbs, coconut milk and olive oil for healthy fats and salt, pepper, cumin and thyme for histamine-lowering herbal action.

Yield: 4-6 SERVINGS

1 cup (240 ml) water

2 medium sweet potatoes

2 tbsp (30 ml) olive oil

1 onion, diced

2 large carrots, diced

1 lb (454 g) lean ground beef

½ tsp cumin

½ tsp dried thyme

½ tsp + a pinch of salt, divided

¼ tsp + a pinch of pepper, divided

1 cup (240 ml) beef stock

1 tsp tapioca flour

¼ cup (60 ml) coconut milk

Fresh parsley, to garnish

Pour the water into the Instant Pot and place the trivet inside. Wash the sweet potatoes and place on the trivet and set to cook with high pressure for 20 minutes. Quick release the pressure and set the potatoes aside to cool.

Drain the water from the Instant Pot and return to the base. Turn on the sauté function and add the olive oil to heat up. Sauté the onion and carrots for 5 to 7 minutes, or until tender. Add the ground beef, cumin, dried thyme, ½ teaspoon of salt and ¼ teaspoon of pepper to the pot with the carrots and onion, and then cook, stirring and breaking it apart with a spatula, until the meat is cooked through. This should take about 10 minutes.

When the meat is cooked, add the beef stock to the pot and bring to a simmer. Ladle out ¼ cup (60 ml) of broth and whisk in the tapioca flour. Then, return to the pot, straining if there are lumps. Stir the meat and allow it to simmer for another 3 to 5 minutes until slightly thickened.

While the meat is cooking, remove the skins from the sweet potatoes and puree the insides with the coconut milk and a pinch of salt and pepper.

The shepherd's pie can be assembled in one large container, such as an 8-inch (20-cm) pan if that will fit into your Instant Pot, or it can be made into 4 to 5 individual serving dishes and cooked in batches. Either way, fill the cooking vessel a little more than halfway with the meat and then use a spoon to spread a layer of sweet potato on top. These are ready to eat like this or they can be reheated in the Instant Pot, covered with foil, on high pressure for 5 minutes, or in the oven under the broiler for 5 minutes. Serve with a garnish of parsley.

PORK AND COLLARD GREENS

Collard greens offer anti-inflammatory benefits and digestive support. They are rich in quercetin, which means that they help lower your histamine levels. Additionally, pork provides an abundance of clean protein and minerals.

Yield: 3 SERVINGS

2 bunches collard greens (10–12 large leaves)

2 tbsp (30 ml) olive oil

¾ lb (340 g) pork tenderloin, cut into cubes

2 cloves garlic, thinly sliced

½ tsp salt

¼ tsp pepper

1 cup (240 ml) chicken stock

1 tsp white vinegar (omit if not tolerated)

Remove the thick center ribs from the collard greens and roughly chop them. Set them aside.

Turn the Instant Pot to the sauté function and pour the olive oil inside. Once hot, sear the cubed pork in batches until browned on all sides, 3 to 5 minutes per side. This can also be done in a cast-iron skillet on the stove.

Add the collard greens, garlic, salt and pepper to the Instant Pot, and toss to combine with the pork. Deglaze the pot with chicken stock and vinegar (if using), scraping the bottom of the pot to release any flavorful bits from searing the pork.

Seal the lid on the Instant Pot and set to cook with high pressure for 15 minutes.

Quick release and serve immediately.

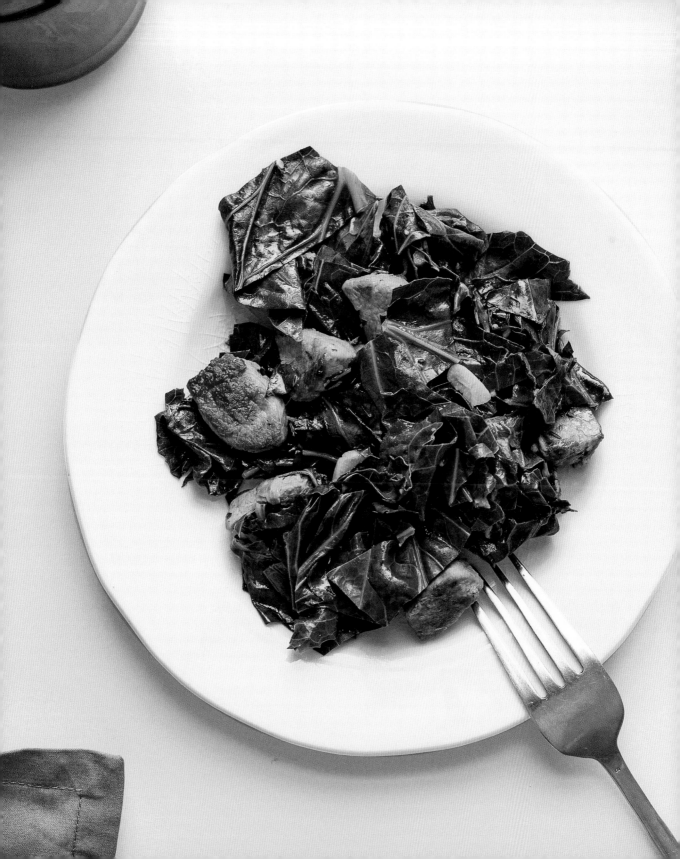

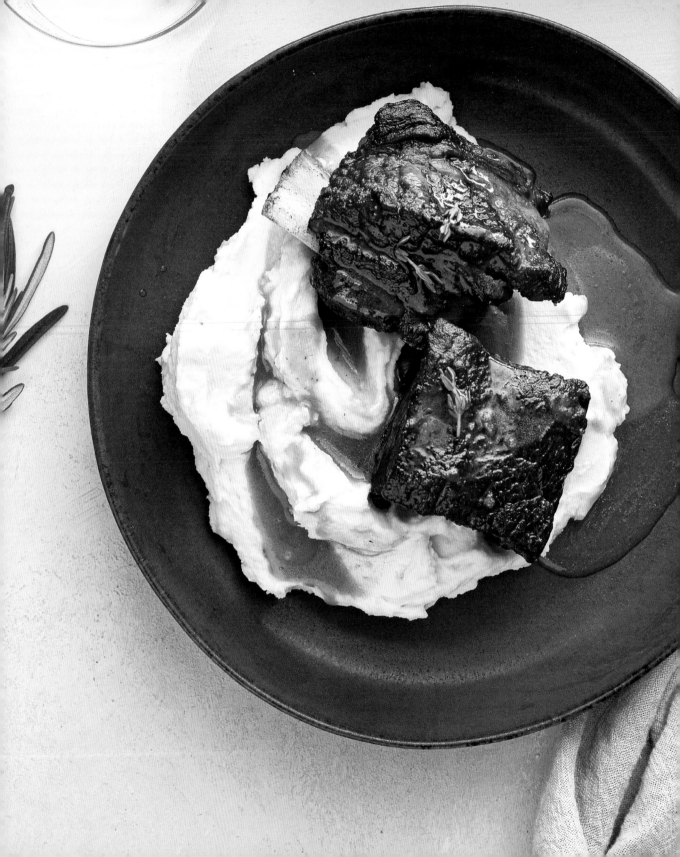

BRAISED SHORT RIBS WITH GRAVY

This is perfect for any holiday or weekend. It's high in protein, and thanks to the peppers, rosemary, thyme, cloves and olive oil, it's also high in quercetin and low in histamine. The butter and olive oil provide plenty of additional healthy fats.

Yield: 4 SERVINGS

2 tbsp (30 ml) olive oil

1 lb (454 g) short ribs

Pinch of salt

Pinch of pepper

1 onion, diced

1½ cups (360 ml) beef stock

4 cloves garlic

2–3 sprigs rosemary and thyme

2 tbsp (28 g) grass-fed butter

1 tbsp (8 g) tapioca flour

Turn the Instant Pot to the sauté function. Heat the olive oil and season the ribs with a heavy pinch of salt and pepper. Working in batches, sear the meat on all sides, 5 to 7 minutes per side.

Return the cooked meat to the Instant Pot with the onion, beef stock, garlic and sprigs of rosemary and thyme. Then, seal the lid and cook with high pressure for 35 minutes.

Quick release the pressure and then remove the meat from the Instant Pot. Switch back to the sauté function, add the butter to the stock and bring it to a boil. Ladle out a small amount of hot broth and whisk the tapioca flour into it to make a slurry. Whisk the slurry into the Instant Pot gravy and allow it to cook for approximately 5 minutes or until thickened.

Serve the short ribs with mashed potatoes or cauliflower and gravy.

MELT-IN-YOUR-MOUTH CARNITAS

Carnitas are a really fun dinner option that also works as a lunch, finger food or side dish. Thanks to all the delicious spices and veggies, it's high in quercetin and low in histamine. Serve it with cauliflower tortillas for a low histamine, gluten-free option.

Yield: 8–10 SERVINGS

2 tbsp (30 ml) olive oil

1 (3–4 lb [1.4–1.8 kg]) pork shoulder, cut into 2-inch (5-cm) pieces

1 tsp onion powder

1 tsp garlic powder

2 tsp (3 g) oregano

1 tsp cumin

½ tsp salt

½ tsp pepper

1 tbsp (15 ml) apple cider vinegar (omit if not tolerated)

1 tbsp (12 g) coconut sugar

1 cup (240 ml) chicken broth

FOR SERVING

8–10 cauliflower tortillas

1 cup (70 g) shredded purple cabbage, tossed with 1 tbsp (15 ml) olive oil and a pinch of salt

1 cup (16 g) cilantro

¼ cup (12 g) sliced scallions

Heat the olive oil on the sauté setting and sear the pork until browned on each side, 5 to 7 minutes per side. Work in batches to avoid overcrowding the pot. Once finished, return all of the seared meat to the Instant Pot and add the onion powder, garlic powder, oregano, cumin, salt, pepper, apple cider vinegar (if using), coconut sugar and chicken broth. Seal the lid and cook with high pressure for 45 minutes. Allow the pressure to naturally release for 10 minutes and then remove the pork from the pot and shred with two forks. Pour some of the cooking juice over the shredded meat and toss.

If you'd like, crisp the pork under the broiler for 10 to 15 minutes, stirring occasionally or in a cast-iron skillet.

Serve with cauliflower tortillas, cabbage, cilantro and scallions.

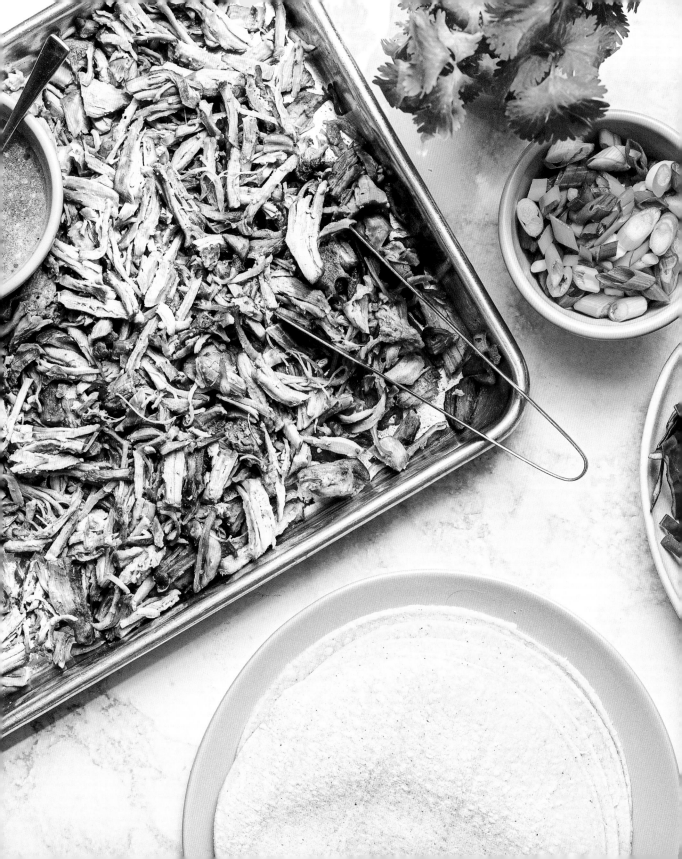

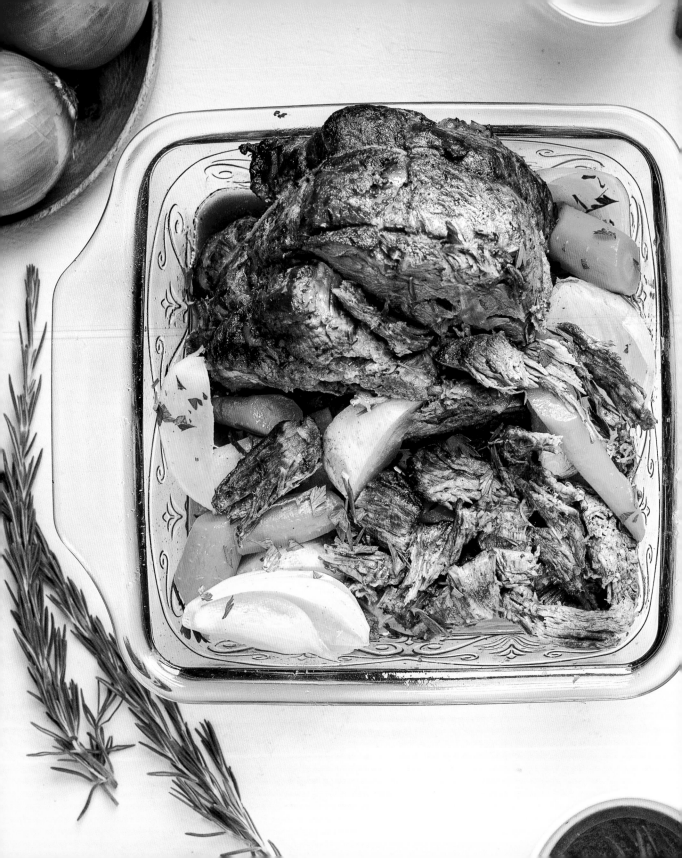

HEARTY POT ROAST

You will love this high-protein pot roast dinner. Thanks to the onion, garlic, salt, thyme, pepper and olive oil, it's a low histamine and anti-inflammatory meal for your entire family to enjoy together.

Yield: 6–8 SERVINGS

1 tsp onion powder

1 tsp garlic powder

1 tsp salt

½ tsp pepper

½ tsp dried thyme

1 (3–4-lb [1.4–1.8-kg]) chuck roast

2 tbsp (30 ml) olive oil

2 cups (480 ml) beef broth

3 cloves garlic

2 sprigs rosemary

2 onions, quartered

2 turnips, sliced into thick wedges

6–8 carrots, cut into 3-inch (7.5-cm) pieces

In a small bowl, combine the onion powder, garlic powder, salt, pepper and thyme. Rub the mixture on all sides of the chuck roast.

Turn the Instant Pot to the sauté setting and heat the olive oil. Sear the meat on all sides until it is a deep golden brown, 3 to 5 minutes per side. Then, add the broth, garlic and rosemary. Seal the lid and cook with high pressure for 1 hour and 15 minutes for a 3-pound (1.4-kg) roast and 1 hour and 25 minutes for a 4-pound (1.8-kg) roast. Once done, allow the pressure to naturally release for 15 minutes, then remove the lid and carefully transfer the roast to a plate to rest.

Add the onions, turnips and carrots, and reseal the lid. Cook with high pressure for 5 minutes and then quick release the pressure. Serve the roast with the vegetables and some broth poured over.

STUFFED CABBAGE SOUP

Cabbage is high in fiber and the amino acid L-glutamine, which means that it supports your digestion. This comforting soup is easy on your gut and low in histamine. It's perfect as a full meal or as a starter.

Yield: 4 SERVINGS

2 tbsp (30 ml) olive oil

1 onion, diced

1 lb (454 g) lean beef

1 tsp salt

½ tsp pepper

½ tsp dried oregano

½ tsp dried parsley

1 red bell pepper, diced

½ head cabbage, roughly chopped into large pieces

3 cups (720 ml) beef stock

2 cups (226 g) cauliflower rice

2 tbsp (8 g) fresh parsley, for garnish

Use the Instant Pot's sauté function to heat the olive oil. Cook the onion for 2 to 3 minutes or until translucent. Add the beef, salt, pepper, oregano and parsley to the Instant Pot and continue cooking, stirring and using a wooden spoon to break the beef into small pieces. Cook for 3 to 5 minutes, or until the beef is browned throughout.

Add the red bell pepper, cabbage and beef stock, and then seal the lid on the Instant Pot. Cook with high pressure for 10 minutes. Allow the pressure to release naturally for 10 minutes, then release the valve and open the lid.

Add the cauliflower rice to the soup and turn on the sauté function. Allow the soup to come to a boil, and then turn off the pot and serve. Garnish with fresh parsley.

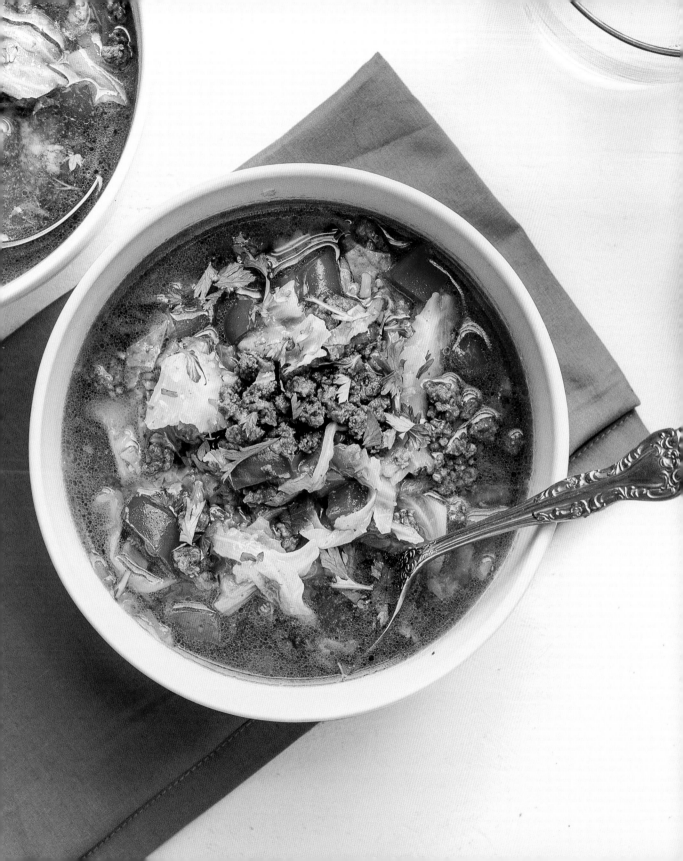

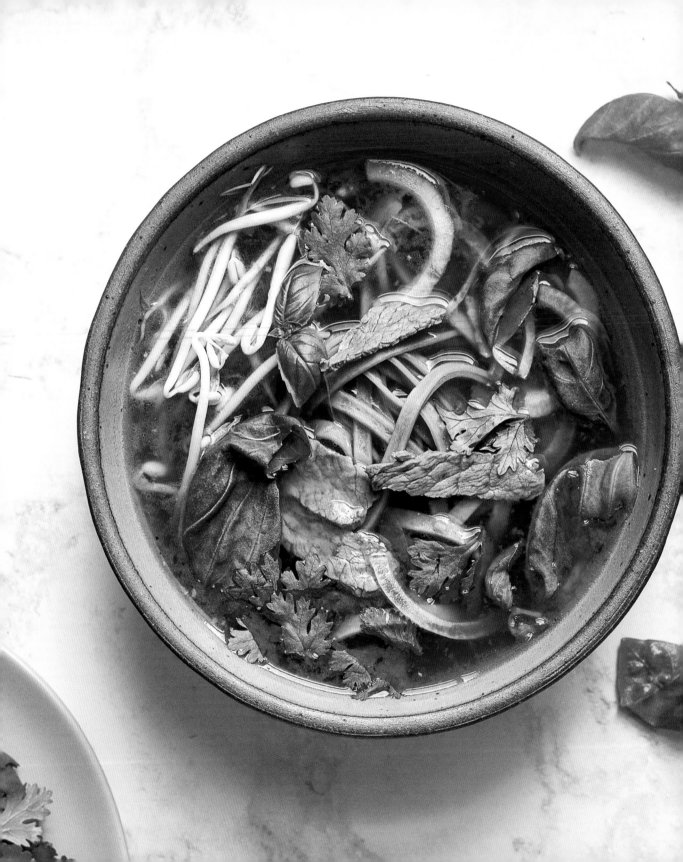

QUICK BEEF PHO

Low histamine cooking is never bland or boring. Just try this Asian-inspired soup. It's Paleo friendly, high in protein and rich in antioxidants. The abundance of herbs helps to reduce histamine, inflammation, pain and the risk of health issues.

Yield: 4 SERVINGS

2 onions, cut in half

1 (2-inch [5-cm]) piece ginger

4 cups (960 ml) beef stock

½ tsp coriander seeds

1 sirloin steak

1 (1-lb [454-g]) package Paleo noodles of your choice

½ cup (57 g) mung bean sprouts

¼ cup (40 g) thinly sliced white onion

½ cup (12 g) Thai or regular basil

½ cup (8 g) cilantro

Char the onions and ginger over a gas flame or under the broiler in the oven. This step can be skipped, but it does add depth to the flavor. Add the charred onion and ginger to the Instant Pot along with the beef stock and coriander seeds. Seal the lid and set to cook for 15 minutes with high pressure.

Meanwhile, place the steak into the freezer to firm up for at least 15 minutes, and then slice as thinly as possible, no more than ¼ inch (6 mm) thick.

Bring a pot of water to a boil and cook the noodles to al dente according to package instructions, then immediately drain and run them under cold water. Drain the noodles and set aside.

When the broth has finished, strain it and discard the onions, ginger and coriander seeds, then divide amongst four bowls. Add a few slices of the thinly sliced raw meat to each bowl—the heat of the broth will cook it. Place some noodles, mung bean sprouts, fresh onion slices and herbs into each bowl.

HEALING CHICKEN SOUP WITH GINGER AND TURMERIC

Soup for dinner? Yes, please. This is an even healthier twist on your grandmother's classic recipe. Ginger and turmeric help to reduce histamine, inflammation, infections and pain, thus making it a perfect choice if you are dealing with symptoms of histamine intolerance or feeling under the weather.

Yield: 4 SERVINGS

2 chicken breasts

3 cups (720 ml) chicken stock

2 ribs celery, sliced

1 carrot, sliced into medallions

1 tbsp (12 g) ground turmeric

1 tbsp (6 g) fresh ginger, minced

½ tsp salt

½ tsp pepper

½ cup (120 ml) coconut milk

1 bunch kale, ribs removed and sliced

Cilantro and parsley, to garnish

Place the chicken breasts, chicken stock, celery, carrot, turmeric, ginger, salt and pepper into the Instant Pot, and seal the valve. Cook with high pressure for 15 minutes and then allow the pressure to release naturally for 10 minutes before opening.

Remove the chicken from the pot and allow it to cool slightly before shredding it with two forks. Meanwhile, add the coconut milk and kale to the pot and turn on the sauté setting. Bring to a boil and allow everything to simmer for a few minutes to soften the kale. Add the shredded chicken back to the pot and then serve garnished with cilantro and parsley.

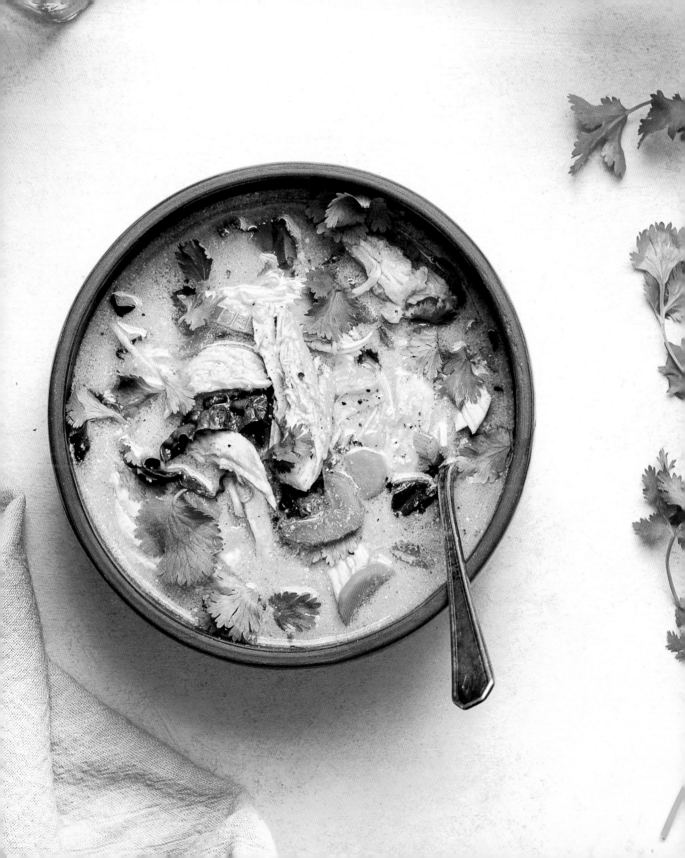

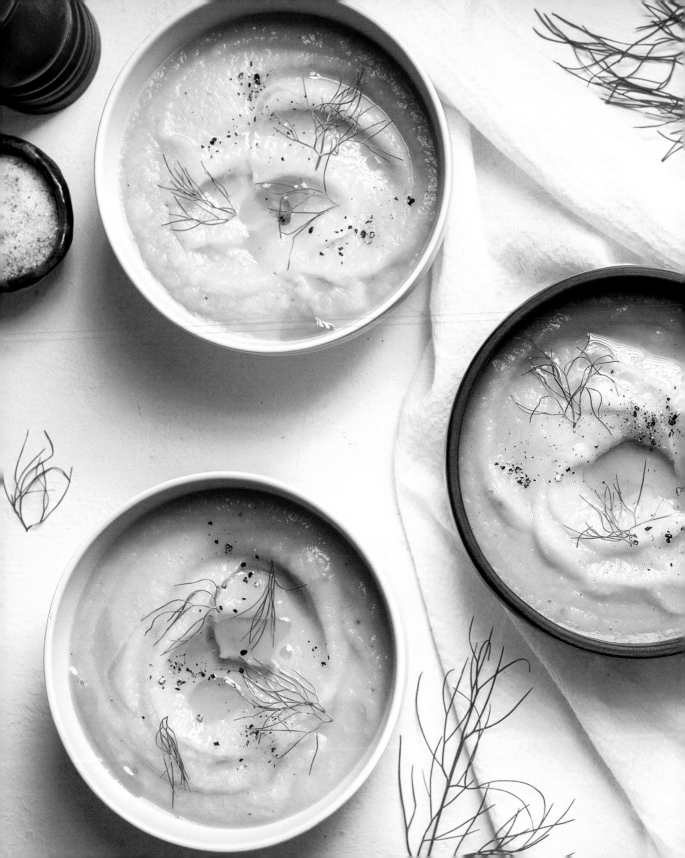

ROOT VEGETABLE SOUP

This soup is another favorite of mine when I am craving a warm soup for dinner made with antihistamine and anti-inflammatory ingredients. The abundance of rutabaga, parsnip, fennel, celery, leek and garlic helps to promote gut health and reduce inflammation.

Yield: 3-4 SERVINGS

½ bulb fennel

2 parsnips

1 rutabaga

1 celery root

1 leek, white part only

4 cloves garlic, peeled and whole

3-4 cups (720-960 ml) chicken or vegetable stock

Salt and pepper, to taste

Olive oil, for serving

Fennel fronds, for serving

Wash, peel and cut the fennel bulb, parsnips, rutabaga and celery root into similar-sized pieces, about 2 inches (5 cm) in size. Cut the leek into 2-inch (5-cm) rings and wash the leek rings thoroughly to eliminate any dirt trapped between the layers.

Place the vegetables into the Instant Pot along with the garlic and chicken stock and seal the lid. Cook with high pressure for 10 minutes and then allow the pressure to release naturally for 10 minutes before removing the lid.

Transfer the contents of the Instant Pot to a blender and blend until pureed, adding more chicken stock if necessary to achieve the desired thickness. You may have to work in batches. Transfer the soup to a large bowl and season with salt and pepper to taste. Serve with a drizzle of olive oil and fennel fronds.

Sides

I love side dishes. A healthy, low histamine side dish will spice up any main dish and provides a great variety to your weekly meals. You may also experiment with serving only side dishes for one meal. These side dishes are also perfect low histamine options for parties and potlucks. The Glazed Carrots (below), Braised Kale (page 106) and Honey Beets (page 108) will fit with just about any meal. But I promise, you will love all these recipes. Even your friends without histamine intolerance will welcome these delicious options at any event.

GLAZED CARROTS

These Glazed Carrots are a simple, low histamine side. Carrots are approved for a low histamine diet and are high in fiber. Thanks to the butter, this side also offers some healthy fats. The thyme, pepper, garlic and honey all offer added anti-inflammatory benefits.

Yield: 3-4 SERVINGS

½ cup (120 ml) + 2 tbsp (30 ml) water, divided

1 lb (454 g) carrots, peeled and cut into 1-inch (2.5-cm) pieces, smaller carrots left whole or halved

1 tbsp (14 g) grass-fed butter

2 tbsp (30 ml) honey or maple syrup

¼ tsp salt

¼ tsp pepper

1 clove garlic, minced (optional)

2 sprigs fresh thyme

Place ½ cup (120 ml) of water into the Instant Pot. If using cut carrots, place them in the steamer basket in the Instant Pot. Otherwise, lay the whole carrots on the trivet. Close the lid and steamer valve and cook with high pressure for 2 minutes. Slow release the pressure for 5 minutes before opening.

Remove the carrots from the Instant Pot and drain the water.

Place the butter, honey, salt, pepper, garlic (if using) and 2 tablespoons (30 ml) of water into the Instant Pot, and use the sauté function to bring the glaze to a simmer. Cook, stirring occasionally until the glaze has thickened, 3 to 5 minutes. Return the carrots to the pot and carefully toss in the glaze, cooking for an additional minute. Transfer to a serving platter, then drizzle with the remaining glaze and top with fresh thyme.

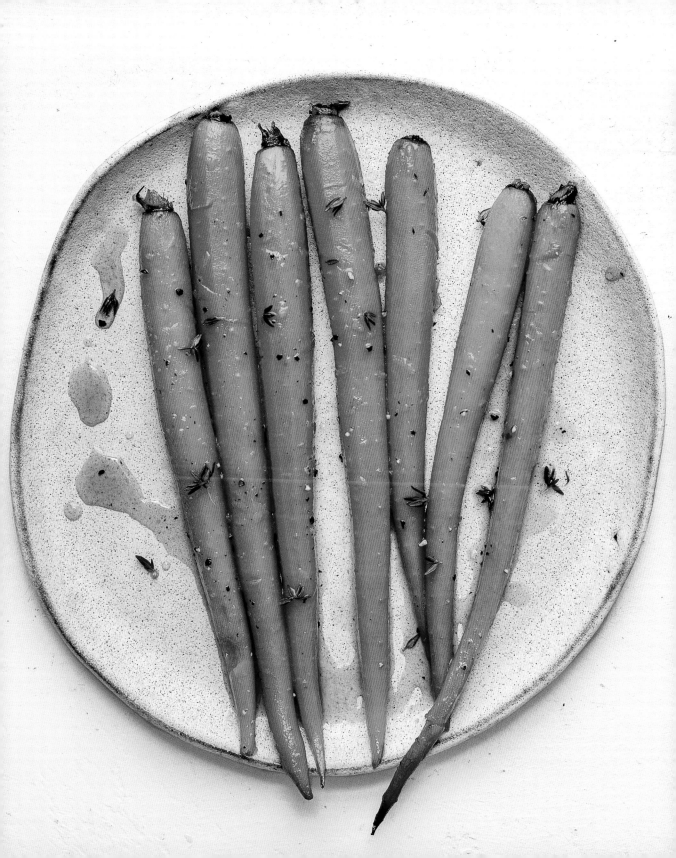

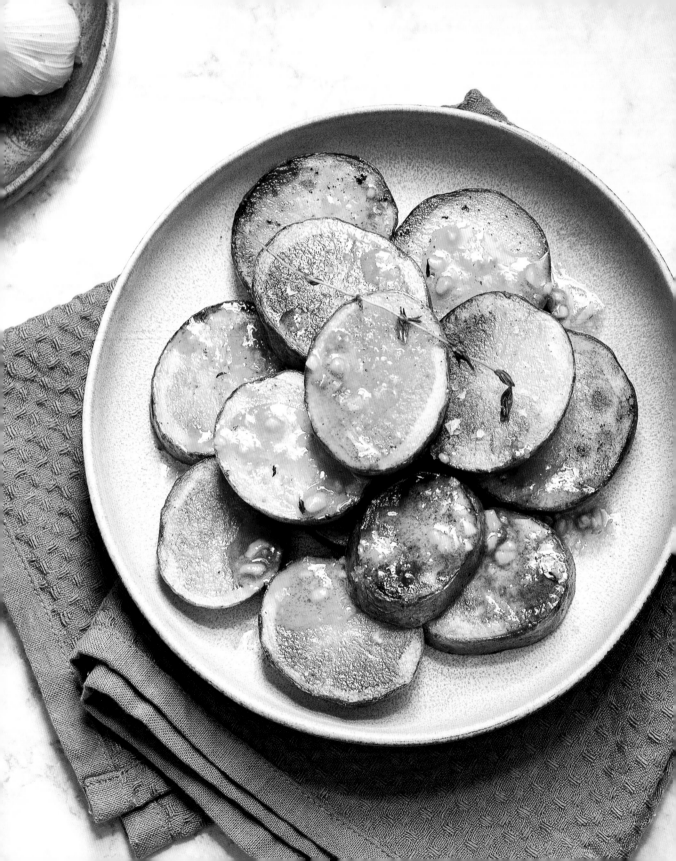

FONDANT POTATOES

Fondant Potatoes are a delicious classic side that your family and friends will love. This side is full of fiber and healthy carbs from the potatoes and healthy fats from the olive oil and butter. Most importantly, this recipe is low in histamine.

Yield: 2-3 SERVINGS

2 large Idaho potatoes, similar in thickness

2 tbsp (30 ml) olive oil

¾ cup (180 ml) chicken stock

1 tbsp (14 g) grass-fed butter

1 clove garlic, minced

Pinch of salt

Pinch of pepper

Wash the potatoes and cut into 1-inch (2.5-cm)-thick medallions. Use a cast-iron skillet or the Instant Pot on the sauté function to sear the potatoes in the olive oil. Cook for 4 to 5 minutes or until they are deep golden brown on each side.

Pour the chicken stock into the Instant Pot and place the trivet inside. Place the seared potatoes into a steamer basket on the trivet—it's fine to stack the potatoes. Seal the Instant Pot lid and cook with high pressure for 6 minutes.

Quick release the pressure and remove the potatoes and trivet from the Instant Pot. Switch to the sauté setting, add the butter and garlic, and bring to a boil. Allow everything to simmer for 3 to 5 minutes, until thickened. Pour the sauce over the potatoes with a pinch of salt and pepper.

BRAISED KALE

Getting plenty of greens is so important to meet your daily micronutrient needs, reduce inflammation, protect your immune system and improve your gut health. Braised kale is low in histamine and anti-inflammatory, and is a perfect side dish.

Yield: 2 SERVINGS

1 tbsp (15 ml) olive oil

3 cloves garlic, sliced

½ onion, sliced thin

1 bunch kale, stems removed and torn into pieces

1 cup (240 ml) chicken or vegetable stock

Pinch of salt

Pinch of pepper

Turn the Instant Pot on to the sauté function and heat the olive oil. Add the garlic and onion, and cook for 1 to 2 minutes. Then, add the kale and stir to mix with the onion and garlic. Add the chicken stock and a small pinch of salt and pepper.

Seal the Instant Pot lid and cook with high pressure for 10 minutes.

Quick release the pressure and carefully remove the kale from the Instant Pot with tongs.

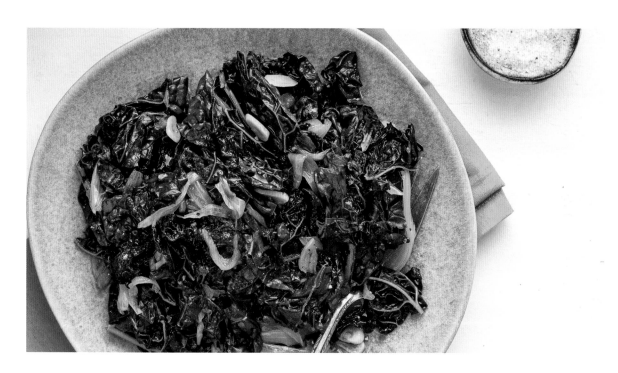

COCONUT CAULIFLOWER RICE

Rice is a commonly enjoyed side dish. The problem is that rice can increase your histamine levels. It is also a common cause of food intolerance. I recommend cauliflower rice instead. It's rich in quercetin and thus helps to reduce your histamine load. It's also a clever way to add more fiber-rich veggies to your meals.

Yield: 2-3 SERVINGS

1 cup (240 ml) water

4 cups (453 g) cauliflower rice

½ cup (120 ml) coconut milk

1 tbsp (15 ml) olive oil

Pinch of salt

Pinch of pepper

¼ cup (4 g) cilantro, chopped

Place the water into the Instant Pot. Put the cauliflower rice into the steamer basket inside the Instant Pot. Seal the lid and set to cook with high pressure for 5 to 7 minutes.

Once finished, remove the rice and transfer to a bowl.

Drain the liquid from the Instant Pot, then turn on the sauté function, and then heat the coconut milk and olive oil with a pinch of salt and pepper. Pour the warm coconut milk over the cauliflower rice and stir in the cilantro.

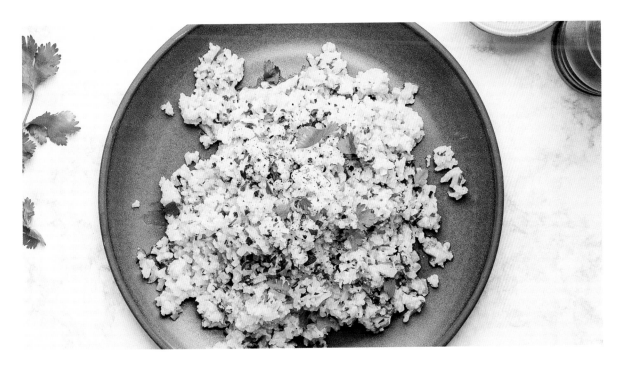

HONEY BEETS

Taking care of your liver is critical if you have histamine intolerance. Beets are the perfect root vegetable to support your liver health and digestion while remaining low in histamine. Honey adds additional anti-inflammatory benefits and some sweetness to the mix.

Yield: 2 SERVINGS

1 cup (240 ml) water

1 bunch golden or red beets (about 4–6), quartered

2 tbsp (30 ml) olive oil

4–6 sage leaves

2–3 sprigs thyme

2 tbsp (30 ml) raw honey

Pinch of salt

Pinch of pepper

Add the water to the Instant Pot and place the steamer basket inside. Place the quartered beets into the basket and seal the Instant Pot lid.

Cook with high pressure for 7 minutes, then quick release the pressure and remove the lid and basket from inside. Drain the water from the pot and return to the base.

Turn on the sauté function and heat the olive oil. Fry the sage leaves for 2 to 3 minutes or until crisped. Add the thyme, raw honey and a pinch of salt and pepper to the pot along with the cooked beets and stir to evenly coat them.

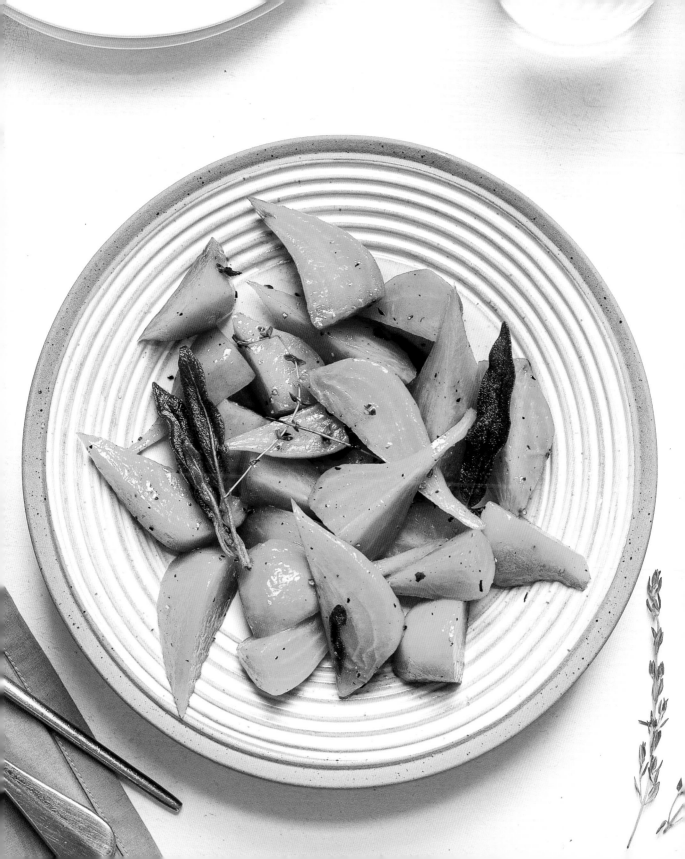

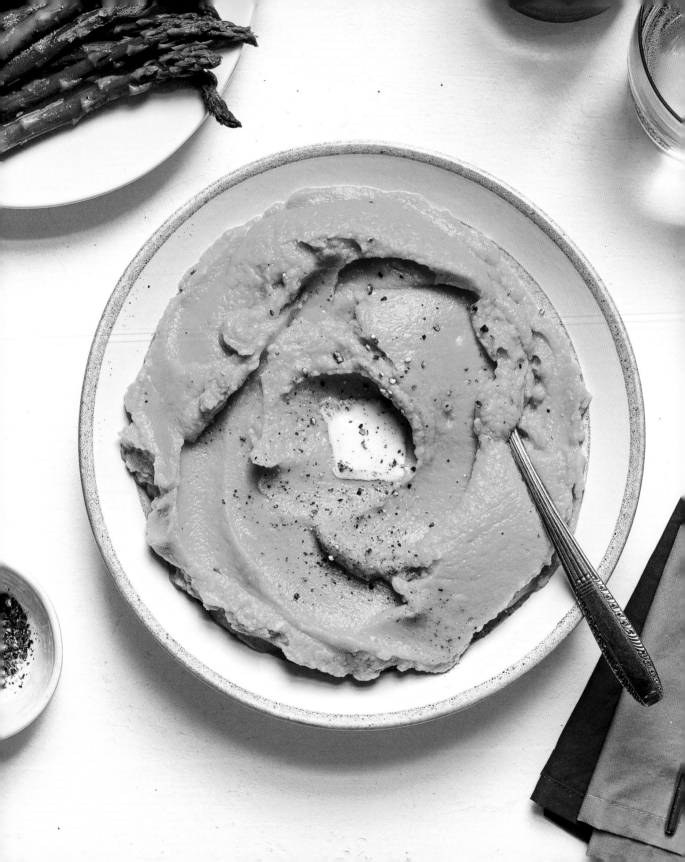

MASHED SWEET POTATOES

This is a creative and healthy twist on everyone's favorite comfort food: mashed potatoes. These Mashed Sweet Potatoes are low histamine, high in fiber, anti-inflammatory, gluten-free and gut friendly. They are perfect for holidays.

Yield: 4 SERVINGS

3 medium sweet potatoes

3 large parsnips

1 cup (240 ml) water

2 cloves garlic

1 tbsp (14 g) grass-fed butter

Salt and pepper, to taste

Peel the sweet potatoes and parsnips, and cut into large, equal-sized pieces, about 3 inches (7.5 cm) in size.

Pour the water into the Instant Pot and place the steamer basket inside. Fill the basket with the sweet potatoes, parsnips and garlic, and seal the lid.

Set the Instant Pot to cook with high pressure for 15 minutes. Once done, quick release the pressure and transfer the contents to a food processor. Pulse the vegetables until you achieve the desired consistency—you can also mash by hand with a potato masher for a chunkier result. Stir in the butter and season with salt and pepper to taste.

GARLIC MASHED CAULIFLOWER

I am starting to question if there is anything cauliflower can't do. It works as an alternative to rice, pizza dough and even mashed potatoes. Thanks to quercetin, garlic and cauliflower both offer antihistamine effects. This recipe is not only perfect for any regular day, but is also a delicious addition at Thanksgiving.

Yield: 4–5 SERVINGS

1 head cauliflower

1 cup (240 ml) water

1 bay leaf

5 cloves garlic

3–4 sprigs rosemary

3–4 sprigs thyme

Salt and pepper, to taste

1 tbsp (15 ml) olive oil, for serving

Roughly chop the cauliflower into large florets, discarding any leaves.

Place the steamer basket into the Instant Pot with the water and a bay leaf. Put the cauliflower, garlic, rosemary and thyme into the basket, and seal the lid.

Cook with high pressure for 8 minutes and then quick release the pressure. Transfer the cauliflower and garlic to a food processor or blender, discarding the herbs and bay leaf.

Puree the cauliflower until smooth and then transfer to a serving bowl. Season the dish with salt and pepper to taste, and finish with a drizzle of good-quality olive oil.

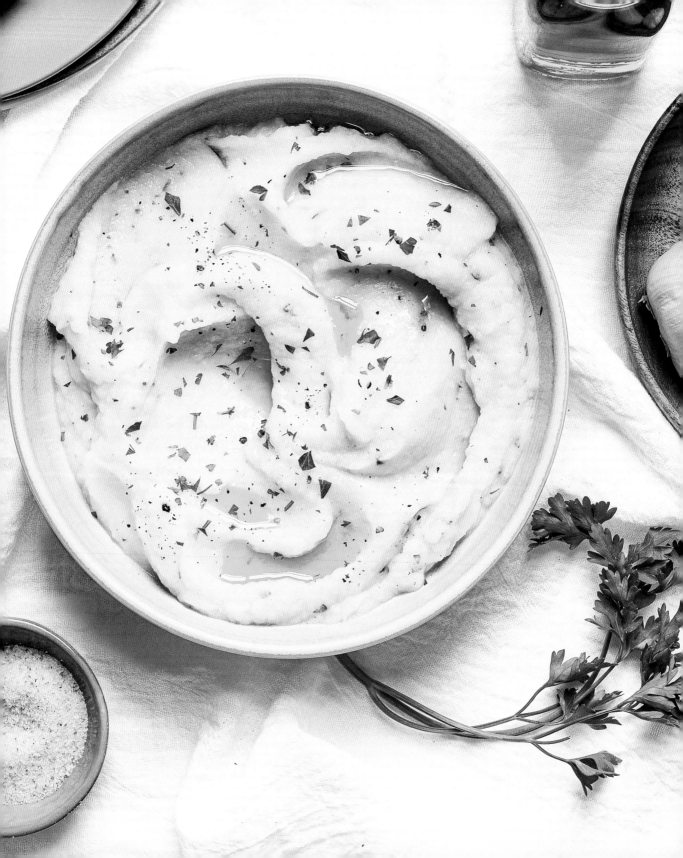

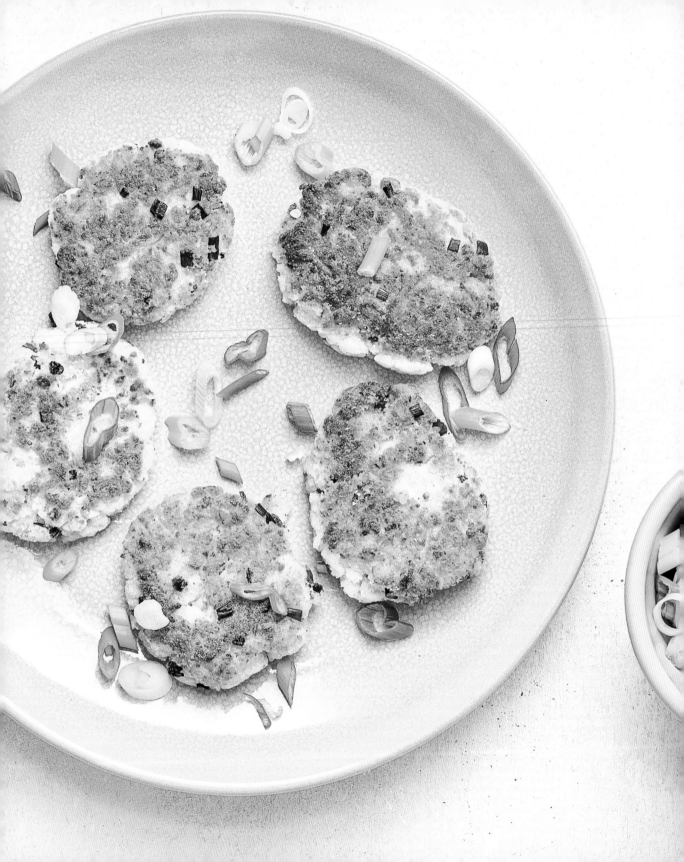

MINI CAULIFLOWER PATTIES

This is another cauliflower favorite. Cauliflower is rich in histamine-fighting quercetin and fiber, offering antihistamine and gut-protecting benefits. It's a great side, starter or snack on any day of the week.

Yield: 6–8 MINI PATTIES

1 cup (113 g) cauliflower rice

½ cup (120 ml) water

3 tbsp (21 g) coconut flour

2 tbsp (17 g) cassava flour

½ tsp garlic powder

½ tsp onion powder

2 tbsp (6 g) chopped chives

¼ cup (60 ml) coconut milk

Pinch of salt

Pinch of pepper

2 tbsp (30 ml) olive oil

1 tbsp (10 g) chopped scallion, for garnish

Place the cauliflower rice into a steamer basket in the Instant Pot with the water in the base. Seal the lid and set to cook with high pressure for 1 minute. Quick release the pressure and then remove the cauliflower. Allow it to cool and then squeeze the water out with a paper towel.

Put the drained cauliflower into a bowl and mix with the coconut and cassava flours, garlic and onion powders, chopped chives, coconut milk and a pinch of salt and pepper, until a dough-like texture has formed. You should be able to squeeze a ball that keeps its shape.

Divide the dough into golf ball–sized pieces and gently flatten them to about ½ inch (1.3 cm) in thickness.

Clean the Instant Pot out and heat the olive oil on the sauté setting. Cook the cauliflower patties until they are golden brown on each side and then transfer to a paper towel–lined plate.

Garnish with the scallions and serve.

SESAME CABBAGE

I love cabbage because it's incredibly high in histamine-reducing quercetin. It's also anti-inflammatory and gut-supporting, and a great way to sneak more veggies in as a side dish. Sesame seeds are a good source of fiber, healthy fats and plant protein, and help to lower inflammation.

Yield: 4 SERVINGS

2 tbsp (18 g) sesame seeds
(omit if not tolerated)

½ head large cabbage or
1 whole small cabbage

½ cup (120 ml) vegetable stock

Pinch of salt

Pinch of pepper

2 tbsp (30 ml) olive or
sesame oil

If using the sesame seeds to garnish, toast them in the Instant Pot on the sauté setting for 3 to 5 minutes, or until golden. Make sure to stir them frequently to prevent burning them. Set the toasted sesame seeds aside to use as a garnish.

Cut the cabbage in half and then cut a "V" shape in the center to remove the core from the cabbage. Cut the cabbage into large wedges, about 2 inches (5 cm) thick. You should get 4 to 5 pieces per half of a large head of cabbage.

Arrange the layers in the Instant Pot—overlapping them is fine—and pour the vegetable stock over them. Sprinkle with salt and pepper, and then seal the lid.

Cook with high pressure for 2 minutes to keep a little bite to the cabbage and up to 5 minutes if you'd like it very tender. Once the cabbage is finished cooking, quick release the pressure and then carefully remove the wedges of cabbage to a serving plate. Drizzle with olive oil and some of the broth, and sprinkle with the toasted sesame seeds, if using.

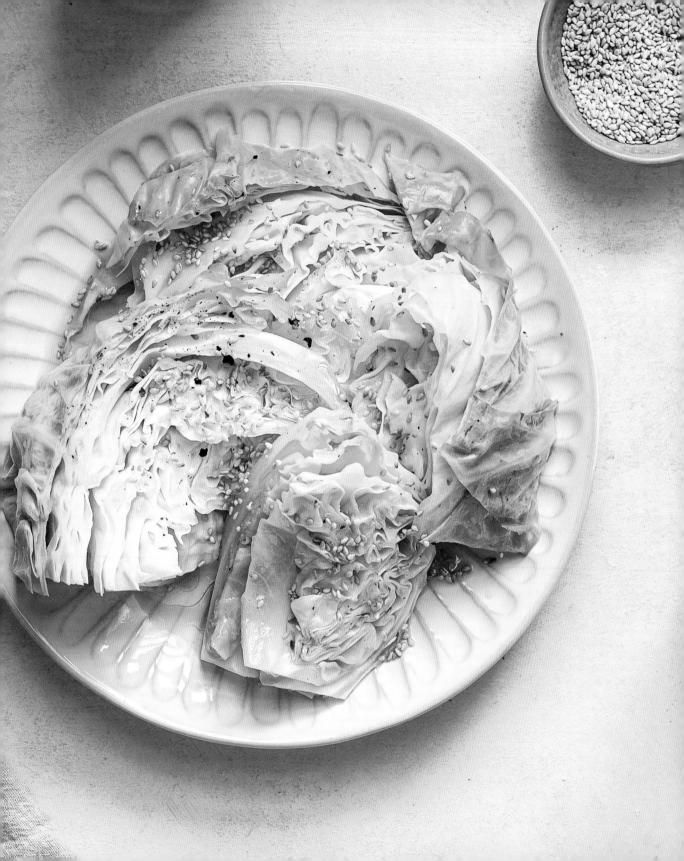

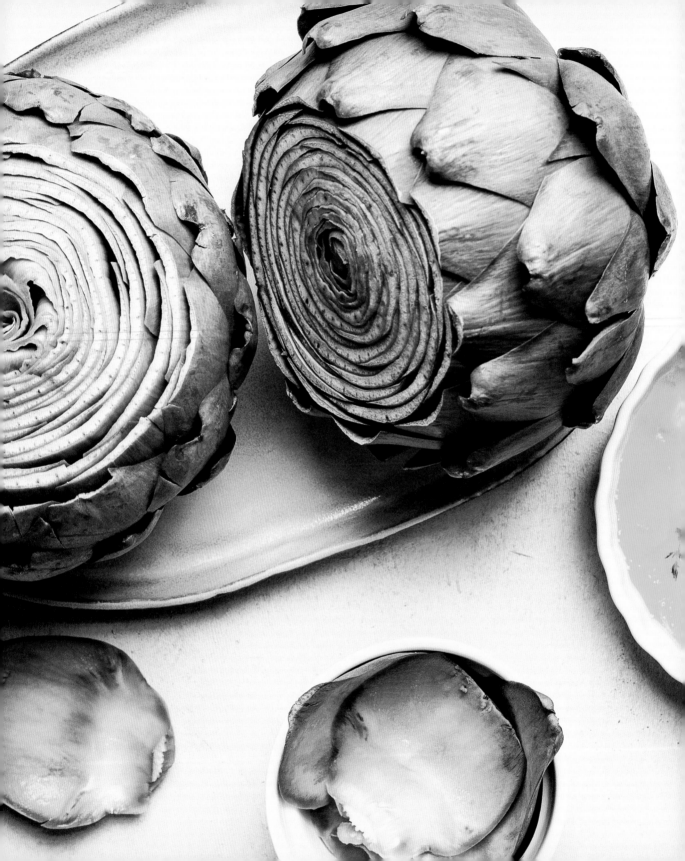

STEAMED ARTICHOKES WITH GARLIC BUTTER

Artichokes are rich in luteolin, an antioxidant that helps to reduce mast cell activation, thus reducing histamine release. Garlic provides plenty of anti-inflammatory benefits and you get healthy fats from the butter.

Yield: 2 ARTICHOKES

2 large artichokes

1 cup (240 ml) water

3 cloves garlic, 2 whole and 1 sliced thin

2 tbsp (28 g) grass-fed butter

2–3 sprigs fresh thyme

Trim the stems from the artichokes, leaving about ½ inch (1.3 cm). Trim the tops off the artichokes and place them on a trivet in the Instant Pot. They don't have to be facing up and can also be cooked on their sides or however they'll fit. Pour the water into the pot and add 2 whole cloves of garlic.

Seal the lid and cook with high pressure for 20 minutes.

While the artichokes are cooking, make the garlic butter by heating the butter and sliced garlic in a small saucepan until the garlic becomes tender, 2 to 3 minutes. Remove from the heat and add 2 to 3 sprigs of fresh thyme.

When the artichokes are done cooking, quick release the pressure and carefully transfer the artichokes to plates. Remove the sprigs of thyme and drizzle the garlic butter over the artichokes before serving.

BROWN BUTTER ASPARAGUS

Asparagus is loaded with nutrients. They help to keep your blood sugar levels steady and keep your histamine levels at bay. Cooking with grass-fed butter adds a dose of healthy fats and flavor.

Yield: 2-3 SERVINGS

1 cup (240 ml) water

1 bunch asparagus, bottoms trimmed

2 tbsp (28 g) grass-fed butter

Pinch of salt

Add the water to the Instant Pot and place the trivet inside. Lay the asparagus on the trivet and seal the lid. Set the Instant Pot to cook at high pressure for 0 minutes. Once the Instant Pot beeps, quick release the pressure and carefully remove the lid and asparagus from inside.

Drain the liquid from the pot and then return to the base and turn on the sauté function. Add the butter and allow it to cook until it is bubbly and beginning to brown. It should smell nutty and fragrant. Pour the browned butter over the cooked asparagus and sprinkle with a pinch of salt.

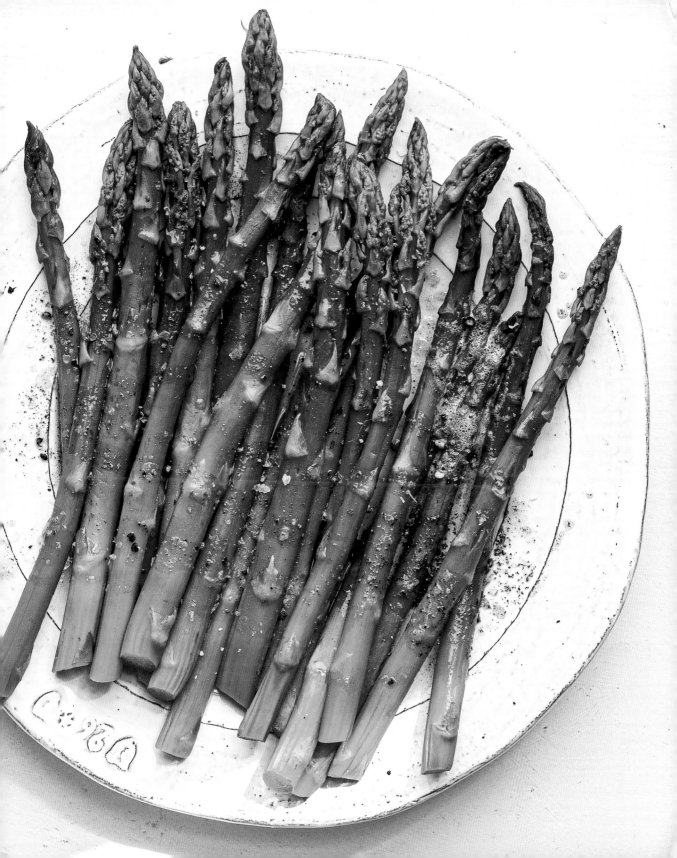

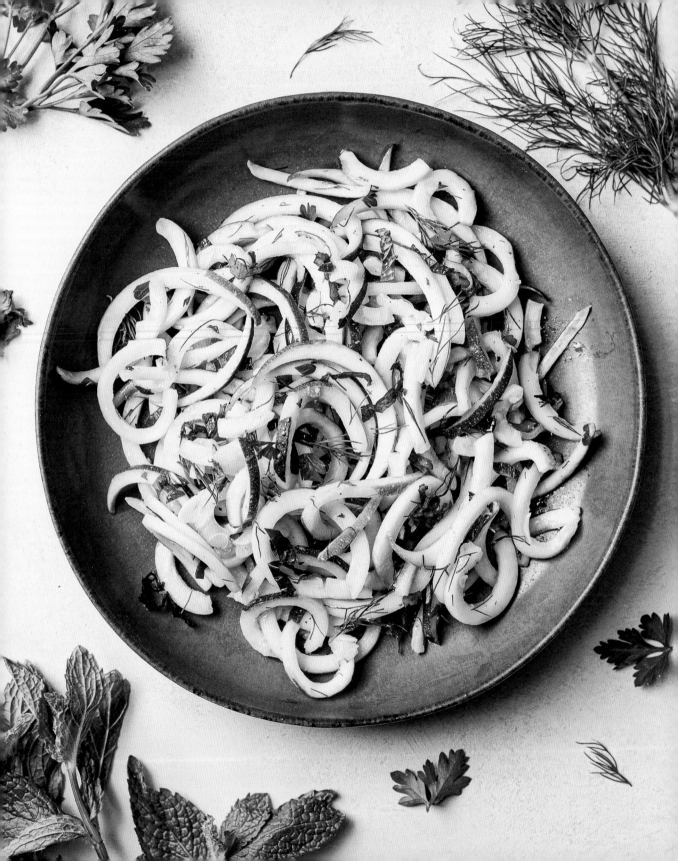

ZOODLES WITH HERB BUTTER

Gluten-filled pasta and noodles are out. Gluten-free veggie zoodles are in. They are easy to make, low in histamine, high in fiber and anti-inflammatory. Served with herb butter, this dish offers some bonus histamine-lowering and anti-inflammatory benefits.

Yield: 2 SERVINGS AS A MAIN, 4 SERVINGS AS A SIDE

2 tbsp (28 g) grass-fed butter

1 lb (454 g) zucchini noodles (from 3 large zucchini)

½ tsp salt

¼ tsp pepper

⅓ cup (32 g) fresh chopped herbs such as mint, basil, parsley and dill

Turn on the Instant Pot sauté function and allow the pot to heat for 1 to 2 minutes.

Place the butter into the pot and let it melt. Then, put the zucchini noodles into the pot along with the salt and pepper. For "al dente" zoodles, cook, tossing often, for only 2 to 3 minutes. For softer zoodles, cook for 4 or more minutes.

Remove the zoodles from the pot and toss with fresh herbs before serving.

ZUCCHINI MEDALLIONS

Zucchini is abundant in nutrients and antioxidants. It's low in histamine and supports your digestion and blood sugar levels. Basil not only has a delicious flavor, but also provides anti-inflammatory benefits to this beautiful side dish.

Yield: 3–4 SERVINGS

2 zucchinis, washed and cut into ½-inch (1.3-cm) rounds

1 tbsp (15 ml) olive oil

¼ tsp salt

¼ tsp pepper

¾ cup (180 ml) water

¼ cup (10 g) basil, cut into ribbons

Toss the zucchini rounds with the olive oil, salt and pepper, then arrange in a 6-inch (15-cm) pan or another pan that will fit into your Instant Pot and cover with a lid or foil.

Pour the water into the Instant Pot, place the trivet on top and put the pan with the zucchini on top of the trivet. Cook with high pressure for 5 minutes. Slow release the pressure for 5 minutes, and then open and garnish with basil ribbons.

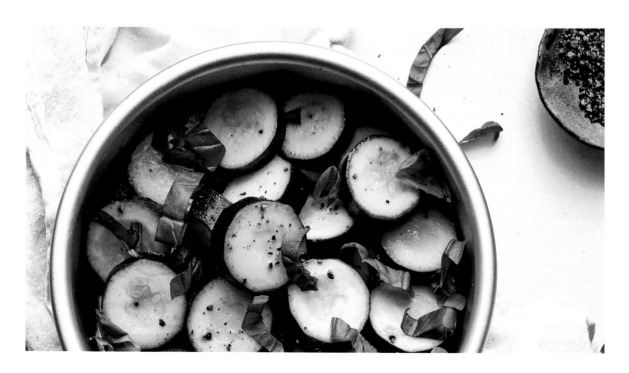

WHOLE HERBY CAULIFLOWER

Cauliflower is every gluten-free person's favorite. It's so versatile. It's rich in quercetin, low in histamine, high in fiber and low in calories. The herbs, salt and olive oil provide bonus histamine-lowering benefits, making this the perfect low histamine side.

Yield: 4–6 SERVINGS

¾ cup (180 ml) water

2 tbsp (30 ml) olive oil

2 cloves garlic, minced

3 tbsp (4 g) minced herbs,
(parsley and cilantro work well)

Pinch of salt

Pinch of pepper

1 whole cauliflower, washed
and leaves removed

Pour the water into the Instant Pot and place the trivet inside.

In a small bowl, combine the olive oil, garlic, herbs, salt and pepper. Spread the mixture over the entire cauliflower and then place it inside the Instant Pot. Cook on high pressure for 3 minutes to retain some bite to the cauliflower and up to 6 minutes for a cauliflower that is tender all the way through. Quick release and serve the cauliflower warm.

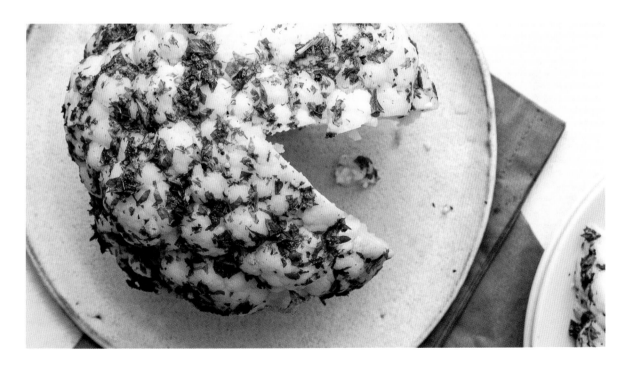

STEAMED SWEET POTATO

Who doesn't love sweet potatoes? They are sweet and delicious. They are also low in histamine and high in fiber. This is a simple recipe with healthy fats from the butter and anti-inflammatory properties from the pepper.

Yield: 2-4 POTATOES

1 cup (240 ml) water

2-4 medium-sized sweet potatoes, washed and pricked with a fork

4 tbsp (56 g) grass-fed butter

2-4 fresh sage leaves, chopped

Salt and pepper, to taste

Pour the water into the Instant Pot and place the trivet inside. Lay the sweet potatoes on top of the trivet and close the lid. With the valve sealed, cook on high pressure for 18 minutes. For smaller potatoes, cook for 16 minutes and for larger potatoes, cook up to 22 minutes. Allow the pressure to release naturally for 10 minutes before opening the steam valve and removing the top. If the potatoes are not tender enough, simply reseal the Instant Pot and cook for a little longer.

While the potatoes are cooking, melt the butter in a saucepan on medium heat. Add the chopped sage leaves and mix. Let the sage cook for 5 minutes while stirring frequently.

Serve the potatoes with sage butter and salt and pepper to taste.

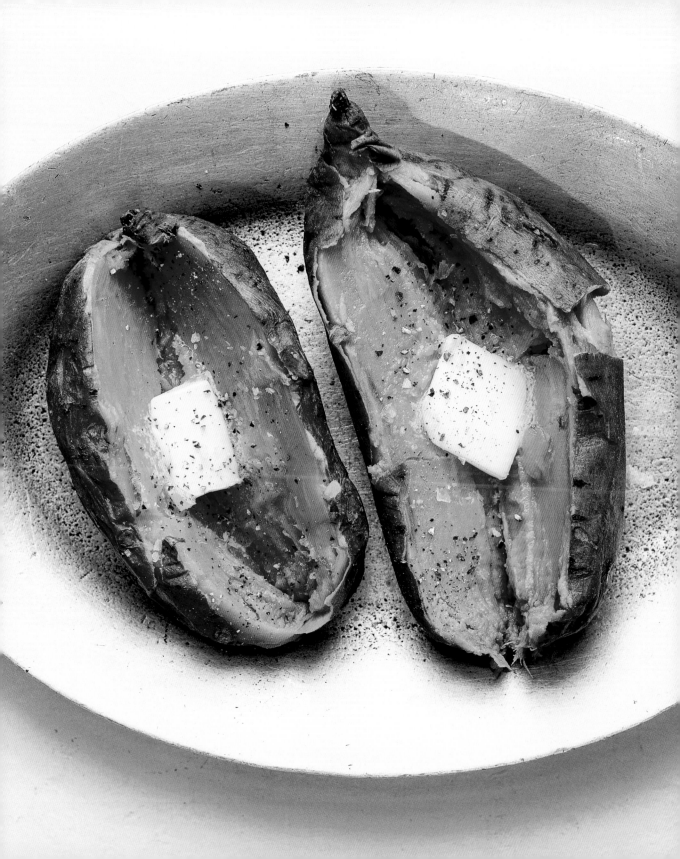

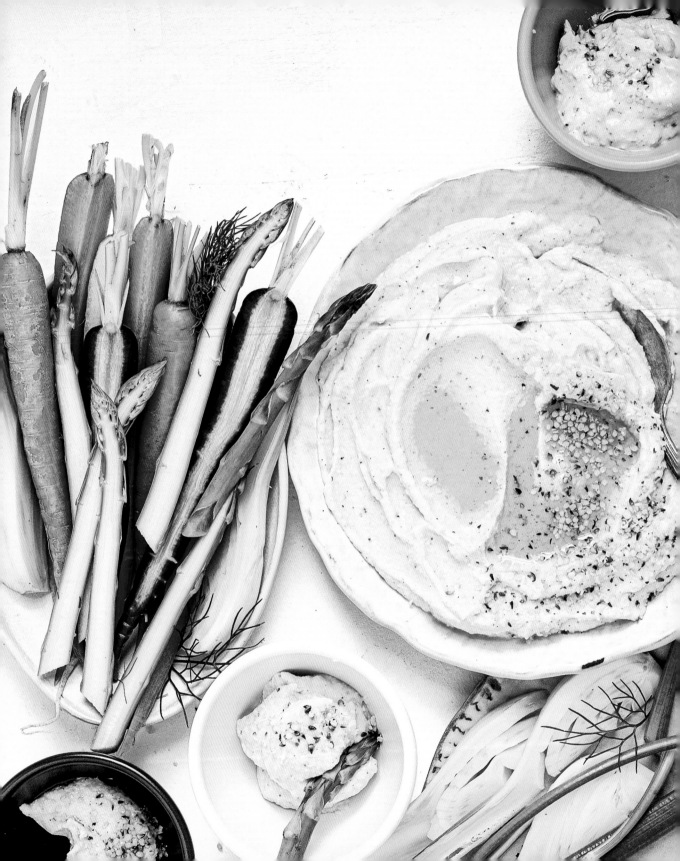

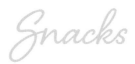

Snacks

There are some days that you just need a snack. Don't deprive yourself.
By choosing these low histamine snacks, you will be keeping your histamine levels down, nourishing your body and satisfying your cravings. Whether you are at work or home, these snacks will help you feel energized and satisfied. Just like my side dishes, these low histamine snacks are also perfect for sharing with your friends and family at parties or potlucks. My friends absolutely love when I bring my Cauliflower Hummus (below) or Sunflower Seed Queso (page 134) to any get-togethers.
They are delicious and are gone in no time.

CAULIFLOWER HUMMUS

This dip offers a unique twist on a Middle Eastern favorite. Cauliflower is high in quercetin, supporting your body with antihistamine power. Dip with some high-quercetin veggies, like broccoli, snap peas or bell peppers, for more histamine-lowering benefits.

Yield: 5–6 SERVINGS

1 cup (240 ml) water

1 head cauliflower

¼ cup (104 g) tahini

¼ cup (40 g) hemp seeds, plus more for serving

2 tsp (10 ml) apple cider vinegar

2 cloves garlic

2 tbsp (30 ml) olive oil, plus more for serving

⅛ tsp cumin

½ tsp salt, plus more to taste

¼ tsp pepper, plus more to taste

Pour the water into the Instant Pot and place the trivet inside. Put the whole cauliflower on the trivet and cook with high pressure for 6 minutes. Quick release the pressure and transfer the cauliflower to a blender or food processor with the tahini, hemp seeds, apple cider vinegar, garlic, olive oil, cumin, salt and pepper.

Process the ingredients until you reach the desired smoothness and taste to see if it needs more salt and pepper. Serve with a drizzle of olive oil and more hemp seeds.

LARGE BATCH GOLDEN TURMERIC MILK

Golden milk is an anti-inflammatory liquid lunch thanks to turmeric and coconut milk. Turmeric is one of the most researched spices for its anti-inflammatory and pain-reducing benefits. Coconut milk is creamy, delicious, anti-inflammatory and histamine friendly.

Yield: 6 CUPS (1.4 L)

4 cups (960 ml) coconut milk

2 cups (480 ml) water

1 tbsp (15 g) coconut oil

3 tbsp (45 ml) honey, plus more to taste

1 tsp freshly ground black pepper

¼ cup (60 g) freshly grated turmeric or 2 tbsp (14 g) ground turmeric

⅓ cup (230 g) freshly grated ginger or 2 tbsp (10 g) ground ginger

2 tsp (10 ml) vanilla extract (optional)

Place the coconut milk, water, coconut oil, honey, ground black pepper, turmeric, ginger and vanilla extract (if using) into the Instant Pot and seal the lid. Heat with high pressure for 7 minutes.

Slow release the lid and open once the valve has released.

Strain and taste. Add more honey, if desired.

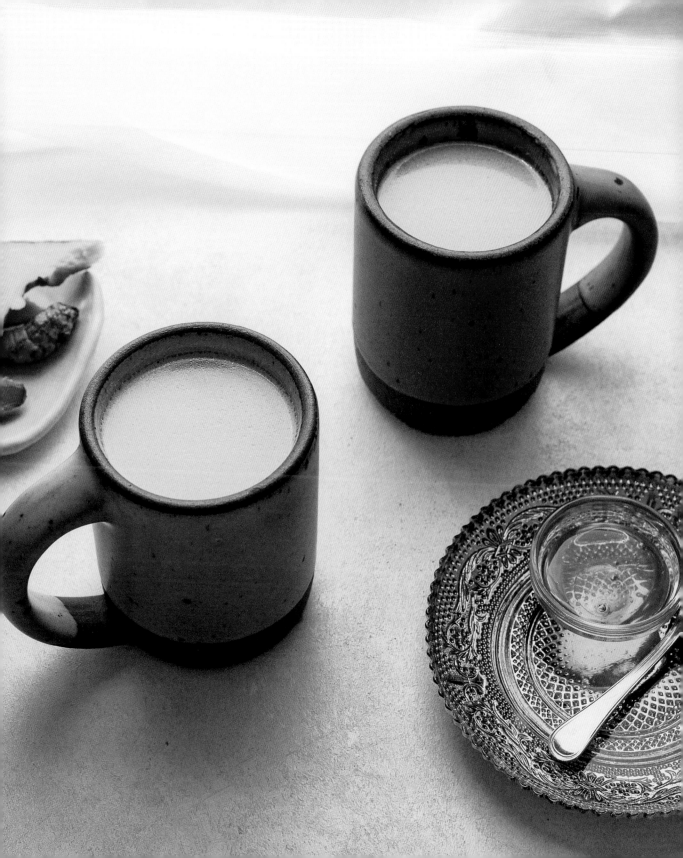

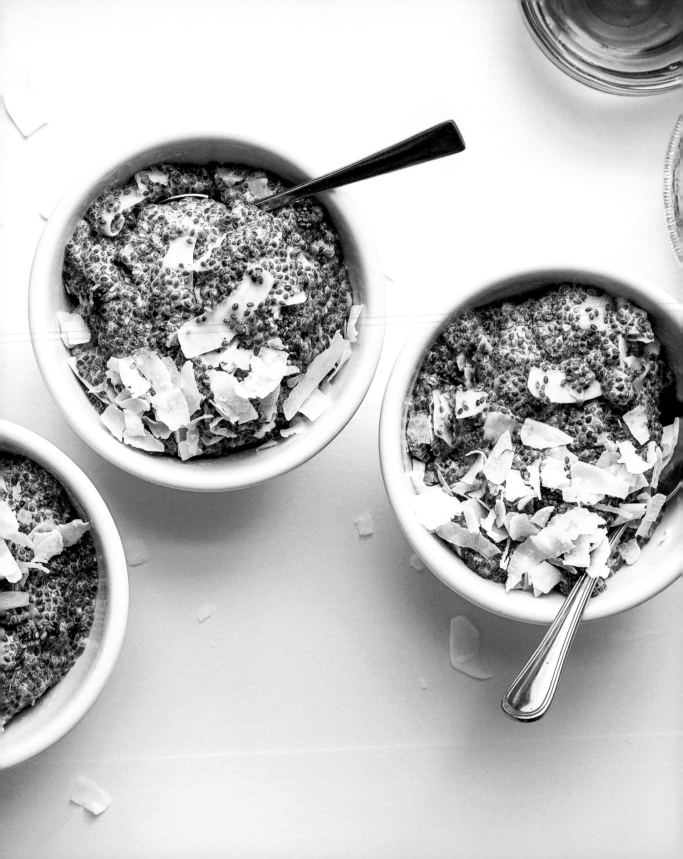

COCONUT CHIA PUDDING

Chia seeds pair perfectly with coconut milk. They create a light yet satisfying low histamine snack, breakfast or dessert. Chia seeds offer bonus anti-inflammatory omega-3 benefits. Add some berries for some antihistamine effects from quercetin.

Yield: 4 SERVINGS

2 cups (480 ml) coconut milk

¾ cup (180 ml) water

¾ cup (122 g) chia seeds

2 tbsp (30 ml) maple syrup

½ cup (47 g) unsweetened coconut flakes, plus more for serving

1 tsp vanilla extract (optional)

Place the coconut milk, water, chia seeds, maple syrup, unsweetened coconut flakes and vanilla extract (if using) in the Instant Pot and turn on the sauté function. Bring everything to a boil, stirring constantly to prevent the bottom from burning and the chia seeds from clumping together. Continue to cook for 2 to 3 minutes until the chia seeds swell and the pudding is thick.

Top with some extra unsweetened coconut flakes and serve warm or chill in the fridge.

SUNFLOWER SEED QUESO

Cheese or queso dips are delicious. The problem is that dairy is inflammatory, histamine-inducing and triggering for many. I recommend this dairy-free "queso" dip instead. The sunflower seeds are a good source of fiber and plant protein, and offer anti-inflammatory effects.

Yield: 4–6 SERVINGS

1 cup (134 g) sunflower seeds

2 small sweet potatoes, peeled and cut into 1-inch (2.5-cm) pieces

½ onion, quartered

2 cloves garlic

1 bay leaf

¾ cup (180 ml) vegetable stock or water, plus extra for thinning

¼ cup (20 g) nutritional yeast (omit if not tolerated)

1½ tsp (4 g) garlic powder

1½ tsp (4 g) onion powder

1 tsp salt

1 tsp pepper

1 tsp turmeric

2 tbsp (30 ml) olive oil

Put the sunflower seeds, sweet potatoes, onion, garlic and bay leaf into the Instant Pot along with the vegetable stock. Seal the lid and cook with high pressure for 5 minutes.

Once finished, quick release the pressure and discard the bay leaf before transferring the contents to a blender or food processor. Add the nutritional yeast (if using), garlic powder, onion powder, salt, pepper, turmeric and olive oil, and process until smooth. Add more water or vegetable stock a couple of tablespoons (30 ml) at a time to reach the desired texture. This works well as a thick dip or a thinner pourable queso texture.

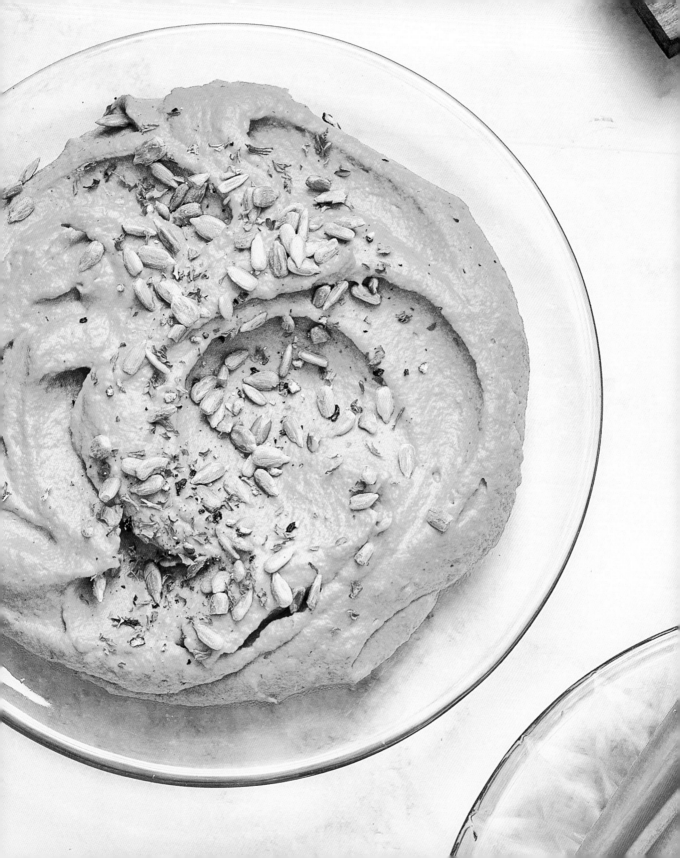

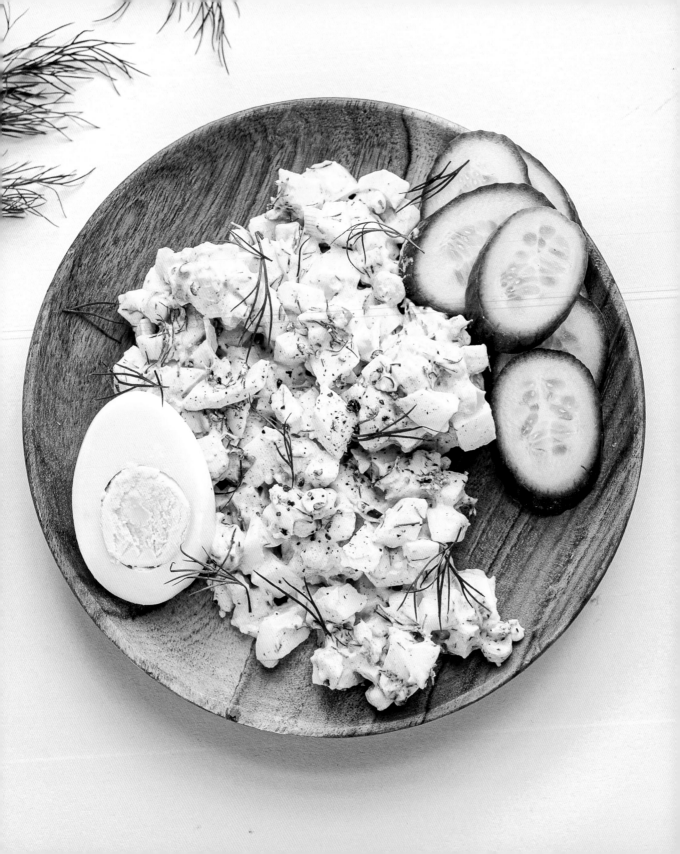

ANTI–INFLAMMATORY EGG SALAD

Choosing an egg salad as a snack is easy and satisfying. Sea salt helps to reduce your histamine levels quickly. Pepper, turmeric and dill offer further anti-inflammatory and antihistamine benefits.

Yield: 3 SERVINGS

1 cup (240 ml) water

6 eggs

¼ cup (60 ml) Low Histamine Mayonnaise (recipe on page 52)

¼ tsp ground turmeric

½ tsp sea salt

¼ tsp ground pepper

2 scallions, sliced

2 tbsp (7 g) fresh dill, chopped

Place the water into the Instant Pot with the trivet inside. Place 6 eggs onto the trivet and seal the lid. Set the Instant Pot to cook for 7 minutes at high pressure. Once finished, quick release the pressure and transfer the eggs to an ice bath.

While the eggs cool, whisk the mayonnaise, turmeric, sea salt and pepper together in a medium-sized bowl, and set aside.

Peel the eggs and roughly chop into small pieces. Gently stir the eggs, scallions and dill into the mayonnaise mixture. Taste and adjust the seasonings as desired.

ANTIHISTAMINE ARTICHOKE DIP

This is a dairy-free twist on a classic dip. Artichokes are rich in fiber, antioxidants, minerals, vitamins and quercetin. They are low histamine, anti-inflammatory and gut friendly. You can share this dip at a party or potluck with your friends and family. It will be an instant favorite.

Yield: 4–6 SERVINGS

1 cup (113 g) cauliflower rice

2 leaves Swiss chard

1 cup (240 ml) water

½ cup (120 ml) Low Histamine Mayonnaise (recipe on page 52)

1 tsp garlic powder

1 tsp onion powder

1 tbsp (10 g) minced shallot

½ tsp salt

1 (14-oz [396-g]) can plain artichoke hearts, roughly chopped

Put the cauliflower rice and Swiss chard into a steamer basket in the Instant Pot with the water in the bottom. Seal the lid and cook for 1 minute with high pressure. Quick release the pressure and remove the steamer basket. Allow the cauliflower and Swiss chard to cool while you prepare the other ingredients.

In a medium-sized bowl, whisk together the mayonnaise, garlic powder, onion powder, minced shallot and salt.

Remove the center ribs from the Swiss chard and chop the leaves into small pieces. Then, add the Swiss chard to the bowl with the mayonnaise along with the cooled cauliflower and the sliced artichoke hearts. Stir well and adjust the seasoning as needed.

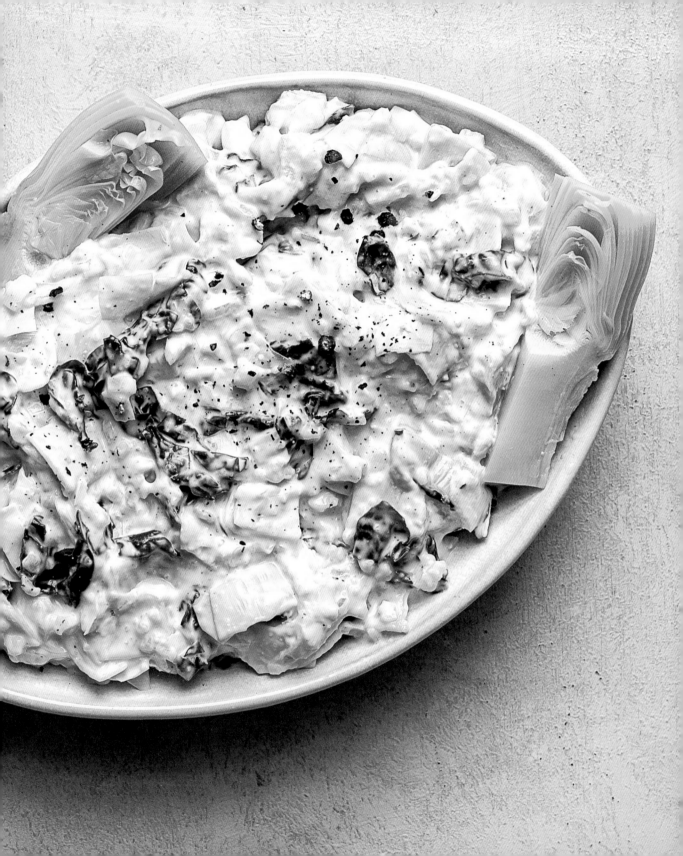

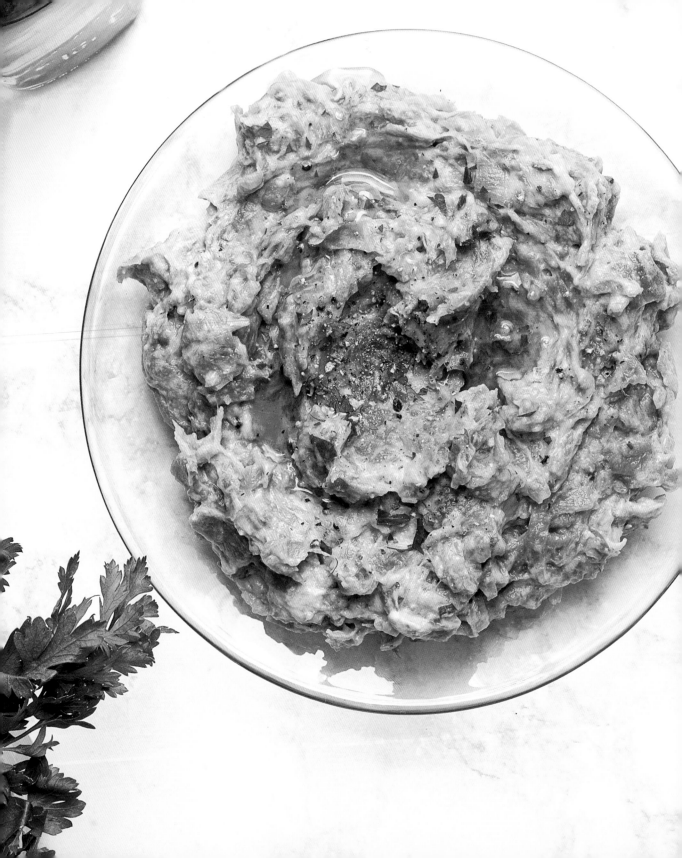

CARAMELIZED ONION DIP

Onions are high in histamine-lowering quercetin, gut-friendly prebiotics, health-promoting antioxidants and anti-inflammatory nutrients. This is a delicious dip to enjoy as a snack or side with vegetables or gluten-free crackers.

Yield: 4–5 SERVINGS

8 medium onions

¼ cup (60 ml) water

2 tbsp (28 g) grass-fed butter

5 oz (140 ml) coconut cream

½ tsp garlic powder

½ tsp onion powder

½ tsp parsley flakes

1 tsp salt

½ tsp pepper

Remove the onion peels, then cut them in half lengthwise and slice them into thin half-moons. Place the onions into the Instant Pot with the water. Seal the lid and cook with high pressure for 5 minutes.

Once finished, quick release the pressure and drain the onions. Return the onions to the Instant Pot and turn on the sauté function. Add the butter and cook the onions for 10 to 15 minutes, stirring occasionally, until they are caramelized. Remove the onions from the Instant Pot and set them aside to cool. This step can be done up to 3 days in advance.

In a medium-sized bowl, whisk together the coconut cream, garlic powder, onion powder, parsley flakes, salt and pepper. Stir in the cooled onions, and then taste and adjust the seasoning as desired.

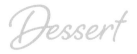

Dessert

Who said that you can never eat dessert on a low histamine diet? Of course you can, as long as you are choosing low histamine options. Feeling deprived is not my style. You will never guess that these desserts are low in histamine. These low histamine desserts are not only healthy and nourishing, but also delicious. They are a perfect treat after a busy day. My personal favorite is the Crustless Sweet Potato Pie (below), while my kids are partial to the Upside-Down Apple Cake (page 145) and Maple Blondies (page 149). Share these treats with your kids, family and friends.

CRUSTLESS SWEET POTATO PIE

This pie is crustless, which means it's also gluten-free. Sweet potatoes provide some healthy sweetness and fiber-rich carbs that support your digestion. It offers anti-inflammatory and low histamine benefits.

Yield: 6 MINIATURE PIES

¾ cup (185 g) sweet potato puree

1 egg

⅓ cup (64 g) coconut or maple sugar

3 tbsp (45 ml) coconut milk

2 tsp (3 g) ground ginger

¼ tsp salt

2 tbsp (14 g) grass-fed butter, melted

1 tsp vanilla extract (optional)

¾ cup (180 ml) water

In a large bowl, whisk together the sweet potato puree, egg, coconut sugar, coconut milk, ginger, salt, butter and vanilla extract (if using) until smooth.

Divide the mixture equally among miniature pie tins or silicone muffin liners. If using regular-sized muffin liners, use only 4 and increase the cooking time by 3 minutes.

Place the water into the Instant Pot and place the trivet inside. Carefully place the miniature pies inside, making sure they remain level. Seal the lid and set the cook time to 7 minutes on high pressure. Once they are done cooking, quick release the pressure and carefully remove the miniature pies. Leave them to rest for a few minutes to allow any steam to evaporate from the tops of the pies. Serve the pies warm or cooled.

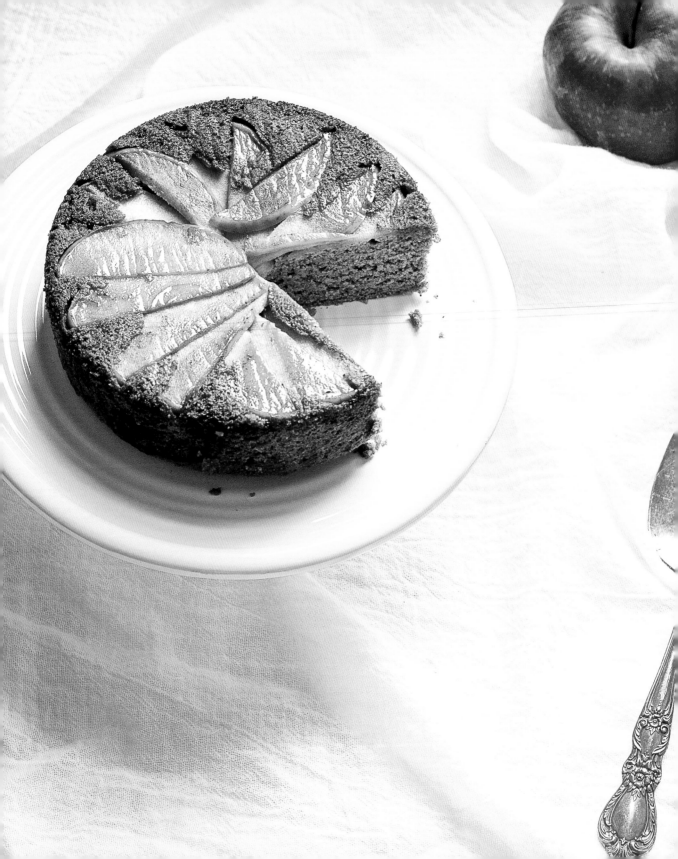

UPSIDE-DOWN APPLE CAKE

I love this Upside-Down Apple Cake. Apples are high in histamine-lowering quercetin. They are also rich in fiber, healthy carbs and micronutrients. This cake is low in histamine and easy to make.

Yield: 1 (6-INCH [15-CM]) CAKE

1 cup (120 g) tigernut flour

¼ cup (28 g) coconut flour

2 tsp (9 g) baking powder

½ tsp sea salt

1 tsp ground ginger

⅓ cup (75 g) grass-fed butter, at room temperature, plus 1 tbsp (14 g) for the pan

⅓ cup (64 g) coconut sugar, plus 1 tbsp (12 g) for the pan

2 eggs, at room temperature

¼ cup (60 ml) + 1 tbsp (15 ml) coconut milk

1 tsp vanilla extract

1 apple, cored and thinly sliced

1 cup (240 ml) water

In a medium-sized bowl, whisk together the tigernut flour, coconut flour, baking powder, sea salt and ginger. Set aside.

Using a stand mixer with a paddle attachment or a handheld mixer, mix together the butter and coconut sugar on medium speed until light and fluffy, for approximately 5 minutes. Add in the eggs, one at a time, scraping the bowl in between additions.

Stop the mixer and add in half of the dry ingredients, then mix on low until all of the ingredients are incorporated. Mix in ¼ cup (60 ml) of coconut milk and the vanilla extract followed by the remaining half of the dry ingredients.

Prepare a 6-inch (15-cm) pan by lining the bottom with parchment. Then, brush the sides and bottom with a tablespoon (14 g) of butter and sprinkle 1 tablespoon (12 g) of coconut sugar inside. Tilt the pan around to make sure the sugar covers the entire bottom and sides. Arrange the apple slices in the bottom of the pan and then pour the batter inside and smooth it out. Cover the batter with foil.

Pour the water into the Instant Pot and then place the trivet inside. Place the apple cake on the trivet and seal the lid. Cook with high pressure for 50 minutes.

Once finished, quick release the pressure and carefully remove the cake. Take the foil off and allow the cake to cool for 5 to 10 minutes before carefully turning the cake over onto a serving plate so that the apples are now on top. Allow it to cool completely before slicing to avoid a gummy texture.

CHUNKY APPLE COMPOTE

Apples are high in quercetin, which means that they help to lower the histamine in your body. Choosing apple compote for dessert offers a low histamine, high-fiber, naturally sweet and spicy option.

Yield: 4–6 SERVINGS

½ cup (120 ml) water

6 large apples, peeled, cored and cubed

¼ tsp salt

¼ tsp ground ginger (optional)

1 tbsp (12 g) coconut or maple sugar

1 tbsp (14 g) grass-fed butter

Place the water into the Instant Pot and then add the apples. Sprinkle with the salt, ginger (if using) and coconut sugar, and then add the butter in 2 to 3 small pieces. Close the lid and seal the steam valve. Cook on high pressure for 1 minute and slow release for 10 minutes before opening the pot. This compote can be served warm or cold.

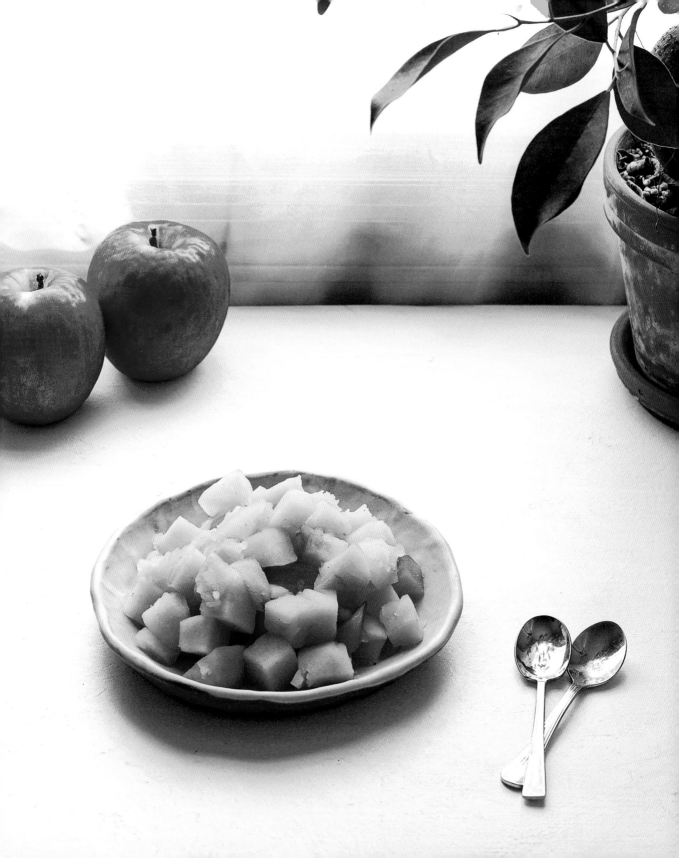

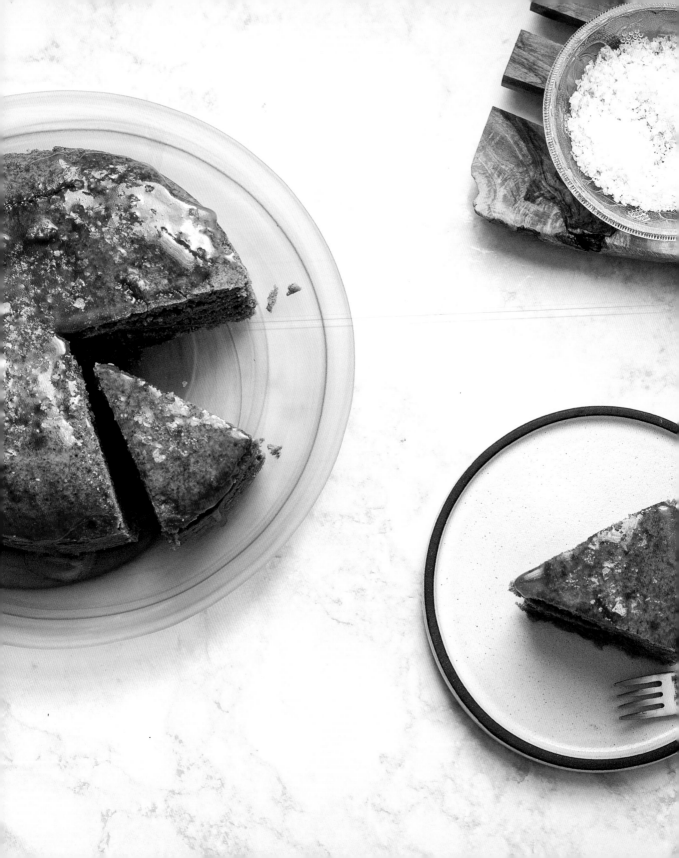

MAPLE BLONDIES

Can you believe that you can eat blondies while on a low histamine diet? It's true. These blondies are the best. They are low histamine, gluten-free and anti-inflammatory. You will want seconds.

Yield: 1 (6-INCH [15-CM]) CAKE PAN

FOR THE BLONDIES

1½ cups (180 g) tigernut flour

½ cup (70 g) cassava flour

1 tbsp (14 g) baking powder

½ tsp salt

½ cup (112 g) grass-fed butter, melted, plus more to grease the pan

2 eggs

½ cup (96 g) maple sugar

2 tbsp (30 ml) maple syrup

1 cup (240 ml) water

FOR THE GLAZE

2 tbsp (30 ml) maple syrup

2 tbsp (28 g) grass-fed butter

Pinch of flaky sea salt

In a medium-sized bowl, whisk together the tigernut flour, cassava flour, baking powder and salt. Set aside. Line a 6-inch (15-cm) cake pan with parchment and brush the sides with melted butter or a cooking spray.

Using a stand mixer or handheld mixer, whisk together the eggs and sugar until the mixture is light. Add in the dry ingredients and mix on low speed until almost fully incorporated, then add the melted butter and maple syrup, and mix until fully incorporated.

Transfer the batter to the prepared pan and smooth the top. Cover the batter with foil.

Pour the water into the Instant Pot and place the trivet inside. Carefully place the pan onto the trivet and seal the Instant Pot lid. Cook with high pressure for 45 minutes, then quick release the pressure and carefully remove the blondies from the Instant Pot. Remove the foil and allow the blondies to cool in the pan, uncovered, to allow the steam to evaporate. Once they are cool, transfer the blondies to a serving plate.

To make the glaze, combine the maple syrup and butter in the cleaned Instant Pot and turn on the sauté function. Allow the glaze to boil for 3 minutes, or until thickened, making sure to stir often so it doesn't burn. Pour the thickened glaze over the cooled blondies and sprinkle with salt.

COCONUT CUSTARD

Going out for custard is one of my favorite childhood memories. You don't have to give up custard on a low histamine diet. Making your own coconut custard offers a dairy-free, low histamine and anti-inflammatory treat.

Yield: 3-4 SERVINGS

1 cup (240 ml) coconut milk

6 egg yolks

¼ cup (48 g) coconut sugar, plus more for topping

Pinch of salt

1 tsp vanilla extract (optional)

1 cup (240 ml) water

In a medium-sized bowl, whisk together the coconut milk, egg yolks, coconut sugar, salt and vanilla extract (if using) and then pour everything through a strainer into a heat-safe bowl. Place the bowl on the trivet inside the Instant Pot and pour the water into the base.

Cook with high pressure for 12 minutes and then quick release the pressure and remove the pudding from the Instant Pot. It should be fully set, but if not, continue to cook for an additional 3 to 5 minutes.

Gently blot any excess moisture from the custard with a paper towel and sprinkle the top with coconut sugar. If you have a blowtorch, use it to caramelize the top, but this step is not necessary.

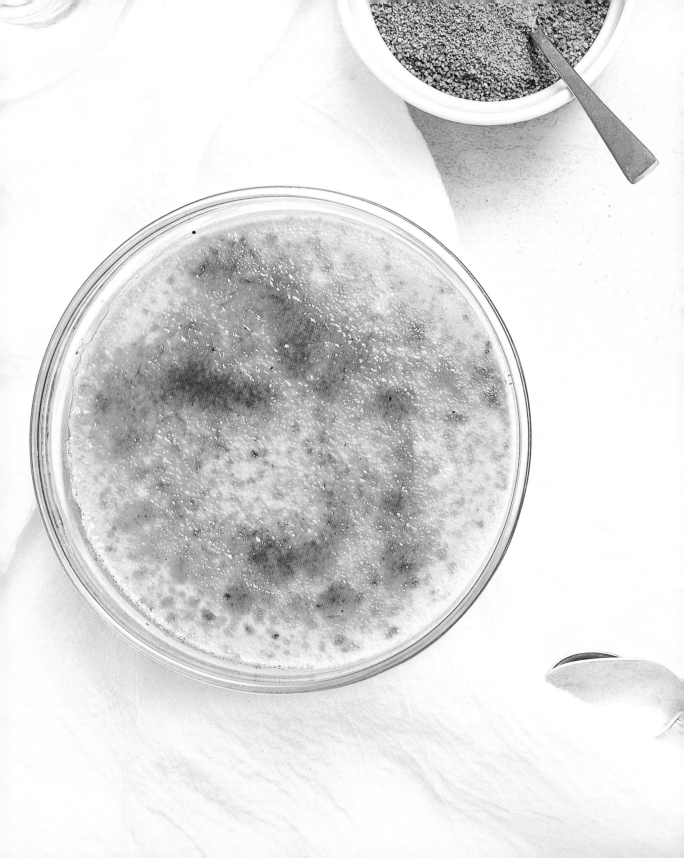

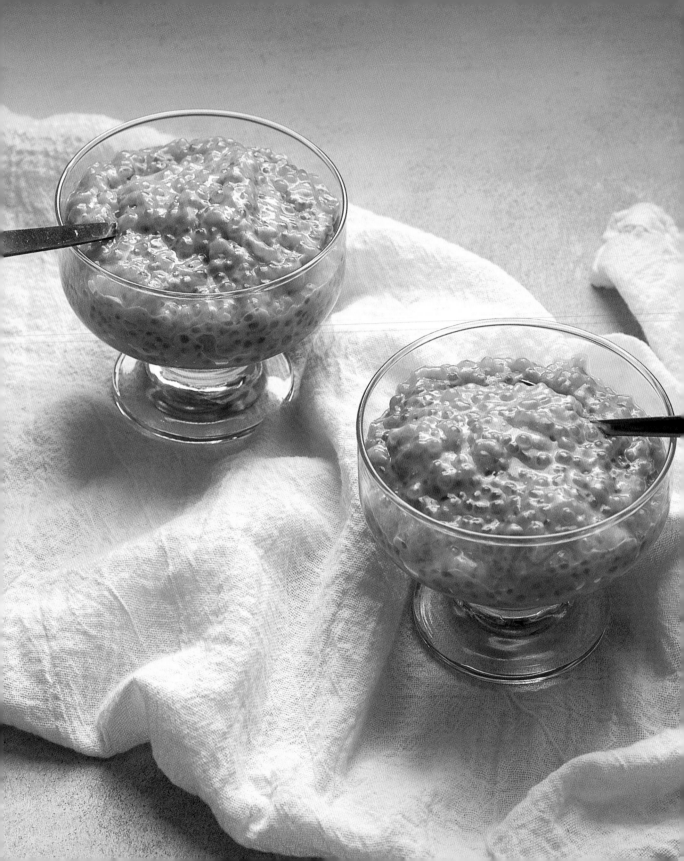

SOOTHING TAPIOCA PUDDING

Tapioca is free from common allergens and is low in histamine. It is loaded with iron and calcium. Choose this tapioca pudding for a low histamine dessert that's gentle on your stomach.

Yield: 3-4 SERVINGS

½ cup (30 g) small tapioca pearls

2 cups (480 ml) water

⅓ cup (64 g) maple or coconut sugar

Pinch of salt

3 egg yolks

¾ cup (180 ml) coconut milk

½ tsp vanilla extract (optional)

Put the tapioca pearls into the Instant Pot along with the water. Seal the lid and cook with high pressure for 6 minutes. Allow the pressure to release naturally for 10 minutes and then remove the lid.

Whisk in the maple sugar and salt, making sure to break up any clumps.

In a separate bowl, whisk together the egg yolks, coconut milk and vanilla extract (if using). Strain the mixture into the Instant Pot and stir well.

Turn on the sauté setting and allow the pudding to come to a boil, stirring constantly with a spatula to prevent burning on the bottom. Cook the pudding until thickened, keeping in mind that it will thicken more once it's cool. Transfer the pudding to a bowl and place plastic wrap directly on the pudding to prevent a skin from forming. Place in the fridge and serve chilled.

STICKY GINGER PUDDING

This Sticky Ginger Pudding is low in histamine, anti-inflammatory, gluten-free and free from common allergens. Ginger is specifically high in anti-inflammatory and histamine-reducing compounds. It's easy on your stomach and so simple to make. You will love it, I promise.

Yield: 2 (4-INCH [10-CM]) MINIATURE BUNDT OR LOAF PAN PUDDINGS

5 tbsp (70 g) grass-fed butter, melted, plus more to brush the pans

3 tsp (15 ml) maple syrup, divided

½ cup (60 g) tigernut flour

2 tbsp (16 g) tapioca flour

2 tsp (9 g) baking powder

1½ tsp (3 g) ground ginger

¼ tsp salt

1 egg

⅓ cup (64 g) coconut or maple sugar

¾ cup (180 ml) water

Flaky salt, to garnish

Prepare two 4-inch (10-cm) miniature Bundt pans by brushing them with melted butter along the base and sides. Pour ½ teaspoon of maple syrup into the base of each pan. It should be just enough to make a thin layer.

In a medium-sized bowl, whisk together the tigernut flour, tapioca flour, baking powder, ginger and salt. Make a well in the center and pour in the melted butter, egg and coconut sugar. Whisk well until everything is incorporated and then divide the dough between the prepared pans. Cover with foil and place on the trivet in the Instant Pot with the water in the base.

Set your Instant Pot to cook with high pressure for 40 minutes and then quick release the pressure and uncover the cakes to release the steam. Allow the steam to evaporate for 5 minutes before inverting the pans and popping the pudding cakes out. Drizzle an additional 1 teaspoon of maple syrup on each cake and top with flaky salt.

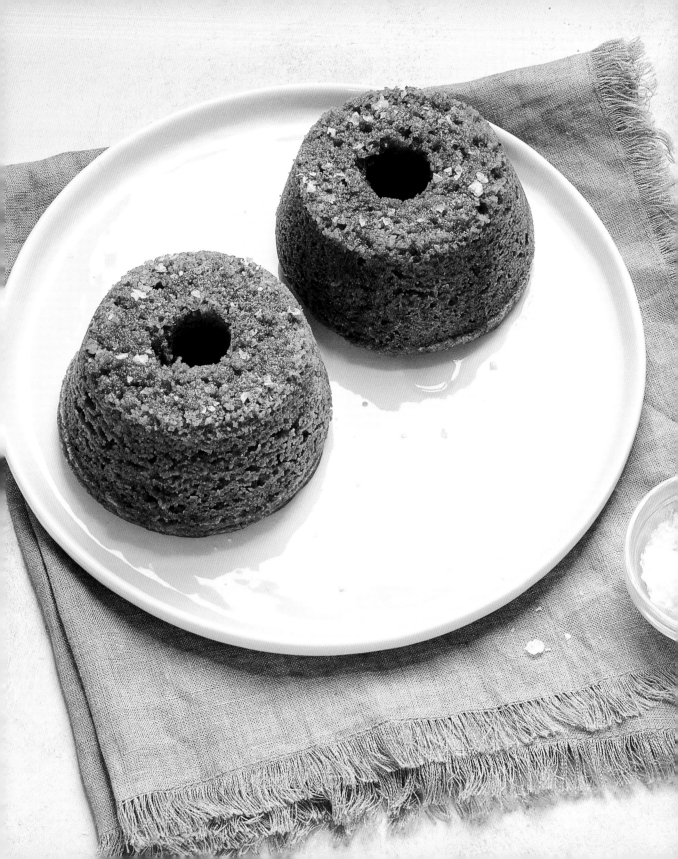

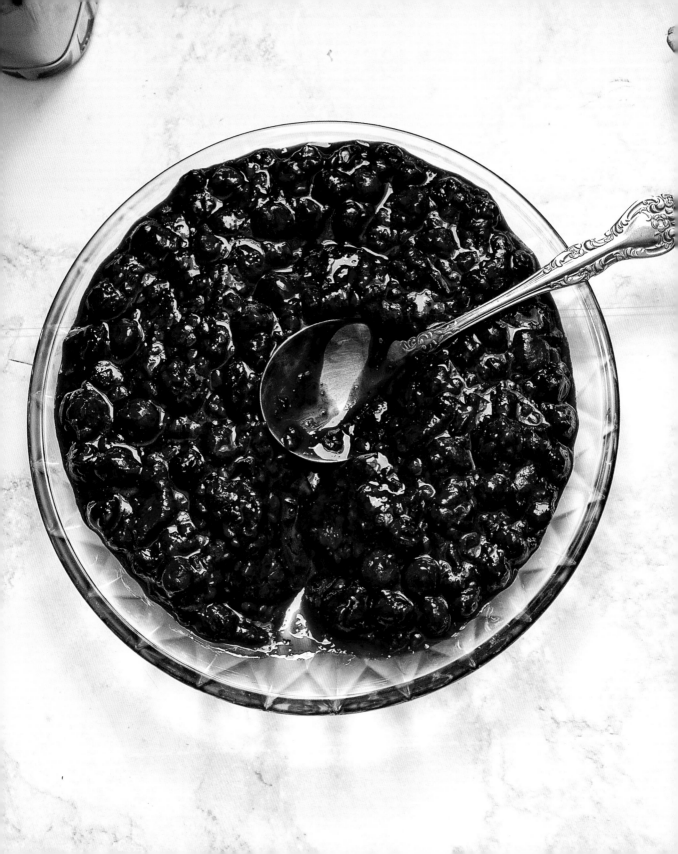

MIXED BERRY COMPOTE

Berries are high in antioxidants and quercetin. Thanks to this berry power, this compote helps to reduce your histamine bucket and inflammation levels while satisfying your sweet tooth.

Yield: 3–4 SERVINGS

3 cups (444 g) assorted berries such as blueberries, blackberries and raspberries (omit raspberries if not tolerated)

2 tbsp (30 ml) maple syrup

1 tbsp (15 ml) water

1–2 tsp (3–5 g) tapioca flour

Place the berries, maple syrup and water into the Instant Pot. Seal the lid and cook for 5 minutes on high pressure.

Once finished, quick release the pressure, remove the lid and then turn on the sauté function. Carefully remove ¼ cup (60 ml) of liquid from the Instant Pot and whisk in the tapioca flour. For a thinner, pourable berry compote, use only 1 teaspoon of tapioca flour. For a thicker jam-like consistency, use 2 teaspoons (5 g). Pour the tapioca slurry back into the Instant Pot and stir to mix. Allow to cook for 3 to 5 minutes until thickened.

BLUEBERRY COBBLER

I recommend anything with blueberries for histamine intolerance thanks to their natural quercetin content. This Blueberry Cobbler is no exception. It's naturally sweet and perfectly healthy without raising your histamine load.

Yield: 4–5 SERVINGS

4 cups (592 g) blueberries

½ cup (96 g) + 3 tbsp (36 g) coconut sugar, divided

1 tbsp (10 g) chia seeds

1 cup (140 g) cassava flour

1 tbsp (14 g) baking powder

½ tsp salt

¾ cup (180 ml) coconut milk

1 egg

Turn the Instant Pot to the sauté setting and heat the blueberries, ½ cup (96 g) of coconut sugar and the chia seeds in the Instant Pot, until the blueberries burst and the juices begin to thicken, for 8 to 10 minutes.

Meanwhile, in a medium-sized bowl, mix together the cassava flour, baking powder and salt. Make a well in the center and add the coconut milk and egg. Whisk well until a dough has formed.

Transfer the blueberries to a 6-inch (15-cm) baking dish and drop spoonfuls of dough around the blueberries. Cover the cobbler with foil and place it on the trivet in the Instant Pot. Cook with high pressure for 30 minutes. Quick release the pressure and then remove the foil to allow the steam to evaporate for 10 minutes before serving. Sprinkle the remaining 3 tablespoons (36 g) of coconut sugar on top of the cobbler to add a bit of a crunch.

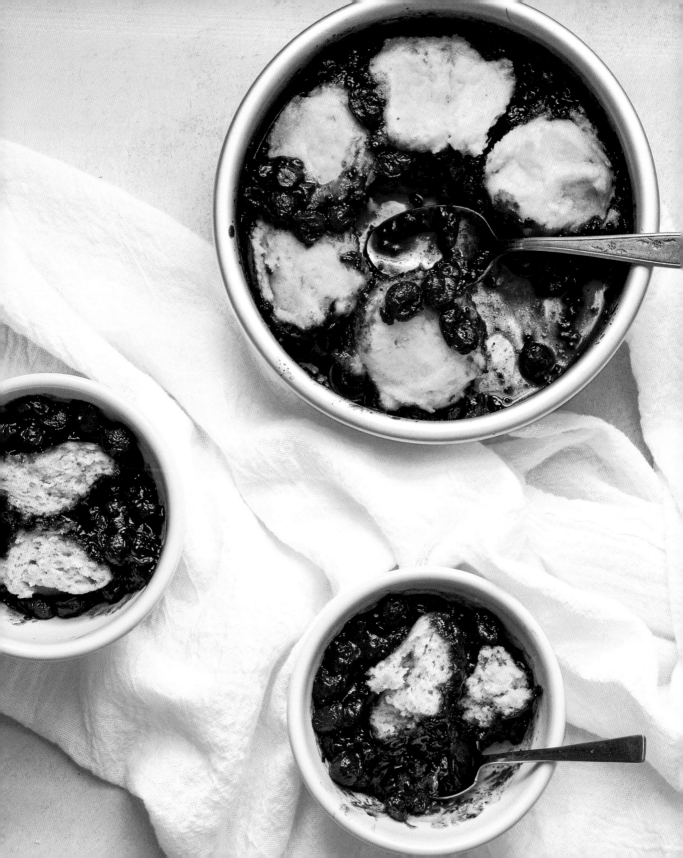

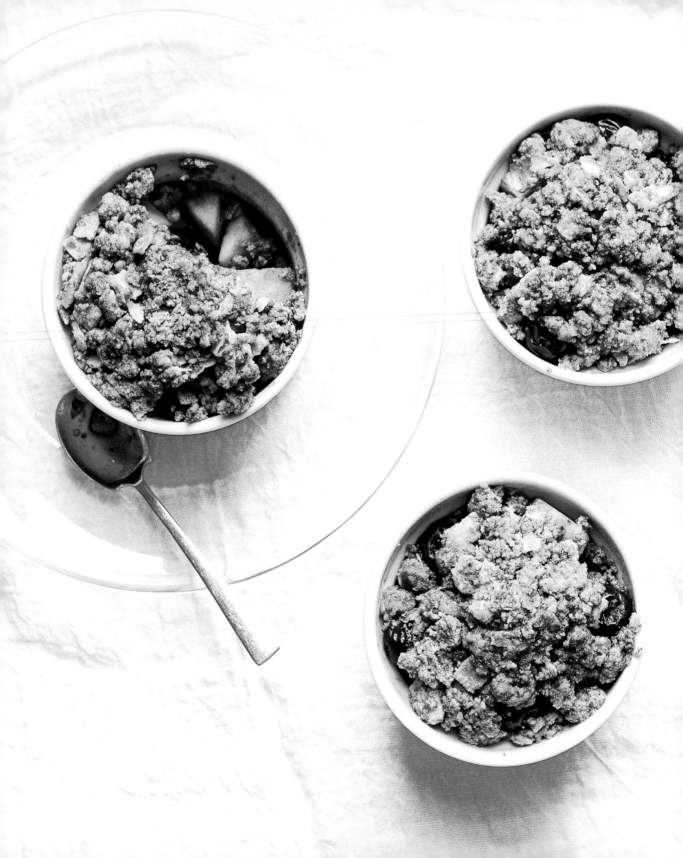

CHERRY APPLE CRUMBLE

Crispy and sweet. What else can I add to this dessert? Cherries and apples are both rich in quercetin to help your body reduce histamine. This delicious baked goodie is dressed up with a crispy crumb topping. It's perfect if you have guests but, of course, you can enjoy it on any weekday.

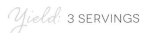 *Yield:* 3 SERVINGS

1 apple, peeled, cored and cut into ½-inch (1.3-cm) dice

1½ cups (231 g) pitted cherries, fresh or frozen

¼ cup (35 g) cassava flour

¼ cup (30 g) tigernut flour

¼ cup (23 g) coconut flakes

3 tbsp (36 g) coconut sugar

¼ cup (60 g) coconut oil, melted

Pinch of salt

1 cup (240 ml) water

In a medium-sized bowl, toss the apple and cherries together and then transfer to a 6-inch (15-cm) pan or divide among 3 individual ramekins.

In a separate bowl, mix together the cassava flour, tigernut flour, coconut flakes, coconut sugar, coconut oil and a pinch of salt, and then sprinkle the mixture over the fruit.

Cover the crumble with foil and place on the trivet inside the Instant Pot. Add the water to the pot and then seal the lid. Cook with high pressure for 20 minutes and then quick release the valve. Uncover the crumble immediately to allow steam to evaporate before serving.

REFERENCES

SOURCES FOR PART ONE

1. Histamine defined. AAAAI. https://www.aaaai.org/Tools-for-the-Public/Allergy,-Asthma-Immunology-Glossary/Histamine-Defined

2. Maintz, L. Novak, N. (2007). Histamine and histamine intolerance. *The American Journal of Clinical Nutrition*, 85 (5), 1185–1196.

ACKNOWLEDGMENTS

TO MY READERS

Thank you for continuing to trust me with your health journey. The amount of support I got on my first histamine book was overwhelming. I hope to continue to provide you with the best resources for histamine intolerance and MCAS. You are doing the hard work to support your bodies and you should feel so proud!

TO MY FAMILY & FRIENDS

Mom, Na and Dad, thank you for continuing to support all of my work and helping me when I need it! Jake, Levi and Liam, thank you for being the most amazing boys any mother could ask for. Lynn, Heidi and Nadine, you are my soul sisters and I love you! Krystal "Pookie Bear" Hohn, thank you for being my partner in work and our podcast, and just for being one of my favorite people in the world.

TO MY PUBLISHING TEAM

Thank you for continuing to allow me to create books that are really helping people. You allow me to put my exact vision on these pages and give me so much freedom to create what I believe is best. You are all amazing and I can't wait for our next project together!

Thank you Lindsey Potter for the beautiful lifestyle photos and Dani McReynolds for help with the food photos.

ABOUT THE AUTHOR

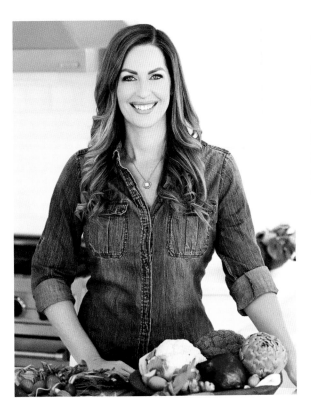

DR. BECKY CAMPBELL is a board-certified doctor of natural medicine who was initially introduced to functional medicine as a patient. She struggled with many of the issues her patients struggle with today and has made it her mission to help patients all around the world with her virtual practice. Dr. Becky Campbell is the founder of drbeckycampbell.com, the host of The Health Babes Podcast and the author of multiple bestselling books, including *The 30-Day Thyroid Reset Plan*, *Long Hauler Road Map: A Guide to Recovery from Histamine Intolerance*, *MCAS and Long Hauler Syndrome* and *The 4-Phase Histamine Reset Plan*. She has been featured on multiple online publications like Mindbodygreen, *Bustle*, PopSugar, *People*, *Men's Health*, *InStyle* and more. She has been a guest on the Mind Pump Podcast, Bulletproof Radio, The Genius Life Podcast and many others as a thyroid health and histamine intolerance expert. Dr. Campbell specializes in histamine intolerance, thyroid diseases and autoimmune diseases, and hopes to help others regain their lives as functional medicine helped her regain hers.

INDEX

A

allergens, 11
almonds: Broccoli Salad, 56
antihistamines, 11
apples
Cherry Apple Crumble, 161
Chunky Apple Compote, 146
Upside-Down Apple Cake, 145
artichokes
Antihistamine Artichoke Dip, 138
Steamed Artichokes with Garlic Butter, 119
asparagus
Asparagus and Dill Soup, 59
Asparagus Frittata, 25
Brown Butter Asparagus, 120

B

basil: Green Minestrone, 68
beans
Almost Niçoise Salad, 55
Green Minestrone, 68
bean sprouts: Quick Beef Pho, 97
beef
Braised Short Ribs with Gravy, 89
Easy Beef Stew with Carrot and Sweet Potato, 78
Hearty Pot Roast, 93
Quick Beef Pho, 97
Stuffed Bell Peppers, 48
Stuffed Cabbage Soup, 94
Sweet Potato Shepherd's Pie, 85
Beets, Honey, 108
bell peppers
Breakfast Hash, 22
Stuffed Bell Peppers, 48
Stuffed Cabbage Soup, 94

Berry Compote, Mixed, 157
Blondies, Maple, 149
blueberries
Blueberry Cobbler, 158
Jumbo Blueberry Pancakes, 35
Mini Blueberry Loaf, 36
Mixed Berry Compote, 157
bowls
Ground Turkey Taco Bowls, 43
Power Veggie Bowl with Carrot-Ginger Dressing, 51
Bread Pudding, Savory Sausage, 26
breakfast
Asparagus Frittata, 25
Breakfast Hash, 22
importance of, 22
Jumbo Blueberry Pancakes, 35
Mini Blueberry Loaf, 36
Nut and Seed Porridge, 30
Savory Sausage Bread Pudding, 26
Scallion Egg Bites, 33
Soft- or Hard-Boiled Eggs with a Twist, 32
broccoli
Broccoli Salad, 56
Power Veggie Bowl with Carrot-Ginger Dressing, 51

C

cabbage
Broccoli Salad, 56
Ground Turkey Taco Bowls, 43
Melt-in-Your-Mouth Carnitas, 90
No-Wrap Pork Dumplings, 47
Sesame Cabbage, 116
Stuffed Cabbage Soup, 94
Cake, Upside-Down Apple, 145
canning jars, 20
carrots
Broccoli Salad, 56

Easy Beef Stew with Carrot and Sweet Potato, 78
Glazed Carrots, 102
Healing Chicken Soup with Ginger and Turmeric, 98
Hearty Pot Roast, 93
Parsnip Soup, 64
Power Veggie Bowl with Carrot-Ginger Dressing, 51
Sweet Potato Shepherd's Pie, 85
Thai-Style Carrot Soup, 63
cassava: Easy Beef Stew with Carrot and Sweet Potato, 78
cassava flour
Blueberry Cobbler, 158
Cherry Apple Crumble, 161
Jumbo Blueberry Pancakes, 35
Maple Blondies, 149
Mini Blueberry Loaf, 36
cauliflower
Antihistamine Artichoke Dip, 138
Asparagus and Dill Soup, 59
Cauliflower Hummus, 129
Coconut Cauliflower Rice, 107
Creamy Cauliflower Soup, 60
Garlic Mashed Cauliflower, 112
Ground Turkey Taco Bowls, 43
Mini Cauliflower Patties, 115
Stuffed Bell Peppers, 48
Stuffed Cabbage Soup, 94
Whole Herby Cauliflower, 125
celery
Chicken Zoodle Soup, 67
Gingery Chicken Salad, 52
Green Minestrone, 68
Healing Chicken Soup with Ginger and Turmeric, 98
celery root: Root Vegetable Soup, 101
cherries
Cherry Apple Crumble, 161
Pork Chops with Cherry Sauce, 81

chia seeds
    Blueberry Cobbler, 158
    Coconut Chia Pudding, 133
    Nut and Seed Porridge, 30
chicken
    Almost Niçoise Salad, 55
    Chicken and Creamy Leeks, 40
    Chicken Zoodle Soup, 67
    Coconut-Poached Chicken, 39
    Garlic Butter Chicken, 70
    Gingery Chicken Salad, 52
    Healing Chicken Soup with Ginger and Turmeric, 98
    The Perfect Pulled Chicken, 44
    tenderloins, 21
    Tortilla-less Green Chicken Enchiladas, 74
    Whole Chicken with Pearl Onions, 82
Chowder, Sweet Potato, 69
cilantro
    Ground Turkey Taco Bowls, 43
    Melt-in-Your-Mouth Carnitas, 90
    No-Wrap Pork Dumplings, 47
    Tortilla-less Green Chicken Enchiladas, 74
coconut milk
    Blueberry Cobbler, 158
    Coconut Cauliflower Rice, 107
    Coconut Chia Pudding, 133
    Coconut Custard, 150
    Coconut-Poached Chicken, 39
    Jumbo Blueberry Pancakes, 35
    Large Batch Golden Turmeric Milk, 130
    Nut and Seed Porridge, 30
    Savory Sausage Bread Pudding, 26
    Soothing Tapioca Pudding, 153
    Sweet Potato Chowder, 69
    Thai-Style Carrot Soup, 63

collard greens
    collard green wraps, 21
    Pork and Collard Greens, 86
compote
    Chunky Apple Compote, 146
    Mixed Berry Compote, 157
Custard, Coconut, 150

D

desserts
    Blueberry Cobbler, 158
    Cherry Apple Crumble, 161
    Chunky Apple Compote, 146
    Coconut Custard, 150
    Crustless Sweet Potato Pie, 142
    Maple Blondies, 149
    Mixed Berry Compote, 157
    Soothing Tapioca Pudding, 153
    Sticky Ginger Pudding, 154
    Upside-Down Apple Cake, 145
diamine oxidase (DAO) enzyme, 12, 15
digestion, 12
dill
    Anti-Inflammatory Egg Salad, 137
    Asparagus and Dill Soup, 59
    Stuffed Bell Peppers, 48
dinner
    Braised Short Ribs with Gravy, 89
    Garlic Butter Chicken, 70
    Healing Chicken Soup with Ginger and Turmeric, 98
    Hearty Pot Roast, 93
    Lamb Shanks with Shallots, 73
    Melt-in-Your-Mouth Carnitas, 90
    Pork and Collard Greens, 86
    Pork Chops with Cherry Sauce, 81
    Quick Beef Pho, 97
    Root Vegetable Soup, 101

    Sausage and Kale Stew, 77
    Stuffed Cabbage Soup, 94
    Sweet Potato Shepherd's Pie, 85
    Tortilla-less Green Chicken Enchiladas, 74
    Whole Chicken with Pearl Onions, 82
dips
    Antihistamine Artichoke Dip, 138
    Caramelized Onion Dip, 141
    Cauliflower Hummus, 129
    Sunflower Seed Queso, 134
dressings
    Carrot-Ginger Dressing, 51
    Honey-Shallot Vinaigrette, 55
Dumplings, No-Wrap Pork, 47

E

eggs
    Almost Niçoise Salad, 55
    Anti-Inflammatory Egg Salad, 137
    Asparagus Frittata, 25
    Breakfast Hash, 22
    Egg Cups with Mixed Greens, 29
    Power Veggie Bowl with Carrot-Ginger Dressing, 51
    Savory Sausage Bread Pudding, 26
    Scallion Egg Bites, 33
    Soft- or Hard-Boiled Eggs with a Twist, 32
Enchiladas, Tortilla-less Green Chicken, 74

F

fennel: Root Vegetable Soup, 101
food prep tips, 20–21
freezing food, 21
Frittata, Asparagus, 25
frozen patties, 21

G

garlic
Garlic Butter Chicken, 70
Garlic Mashed Cauliflower, 112
Steamed Artichokes with
Garlic Butter, 119
ginger
Gingery Chicken Salad, 52
Healing Chicken Soup with
Ginger and Turmeric, 98
Large Batch Golden
Turmeric Milk, 130
Power Veggie Bowl with
Carrot-Ginger Dressing, 51
Sticky Ginger Pudding, 154
Thai-Style Carrot Soup, 63
Golden Turmeric Milk, Large
Batch, 130
grapes: Gingery Chicken Salad,
52
green beans
Almost Niçoise Salad, 55
Green Minestrone, 68
greens
Almost Niçoise Salad, 55
Antihistamine Artichoke Dip,
138
Braised Kale, 106
Egg Cups with Mixed
Greens, 29
Ground Turkey Taco Bowls,
43
Healing Chicken Soup with
Ginger and Turmeric, 98
Pork and Collard Greens, 86
Power Veggie Bowl with
Carrot-Ginger Dressing, 51
Sausage and Kale Stew, 77
Savory Sausage Bread
Pudding, 26
grocery shopping, 20

H

Hash, Breakfast, 22
hemp seeds
Cauliflower Hummus, 129

Power Veggie Bowl with
Carrot-Ginger Dressing, 51
histamine, 11–12
histamine intolerance
about, 11–12
causes of, 14–15
low histamine diet for, 15–16
personal story of, 9
symptoms of, 12–13
histamine N-methyltransferase
(HNMT), 12
honey
Honey Beets, 108
Honey-Shallot Vinaigrette,
55
Large Batch Golden
Turmeric Milk, 130
Hummus, Cauliflower, 129
hydrochloric acid, 12

I

immune system, 11
inflammation, 16
Instant Pot
cooking with, 19–21
food prep tips, 20–21

K

kale
Braised Kale, 106
Egg Cups with Mixed
Greens, 29
Healing Chicken Soup with
Ginger and Turmeric, 98
Sausage and Kale Stew, 77

L

lamb
Lamb Shanks with Shallots,
73
Stuffed Bell Peppers, 48

leeks
Chicken and Creamy Leeks,
40
Creamy Cauliflower Soup,
60
Root Vegetable Soup, 101
leftovers, 21
low histamine diet, 15–17
lunch
Almost Niçoise Salad, 55
Asparagus and Dill Soup,
59
Broccoli Salad, 56
Chicken and Creamy Leeks,
40
Chicken Zoodle Soup, 67
Coconut-Poached Chicken,
39
Creamy Cauliflower Soup,
60
Gingery Chicken Salad, 52
Green Minestrone, 68
Ground Turkey Taco Bowls,
43
importance of, 39
No-Wrap Pork Dumplings,
47
Parsnip Soup, 64
The Perfect Pulled Chicken,
44
Power Veggie Bowl with
Carrot-Ginger Dressing, 51
Stuffed Bell Peppers, 48
Sweet Potato Chowder, 69
Thai-Style Carrot Soup, 63

M

Maple Blondies, 149
Mayonnaise, Low Histamine, 52
meal plans, 20
microgreens: Ground Turkey
Taco Bowls, 43
Minestrone, Green, 68
mung bean sprouts: Quick Beef
Pho, 97
mustard greens: Egg Cups with
Mixed Greens, 29

N

neurotransmitters, 12
noodles: Quick Beef Pho, 97
nutritional yeast
    Creamy Cauliflower Soup, 60
    Sunflower Seed Queso, 134
nuts and seeds
    Broccoli Salad, 56
    Cauliflower Hummus, 129
    Nut and Seed Porridge, 30
    Power Veggie Bowl with
      Carrot-Ginger Dressing, 51
    Sesame Cabbage, 116
    Sunflower Seed Queso, 134

O

onion
    Breakfast Hash, 22
    Broccoli Salad, 56
    Caramelized Onion Dip, 141
    Chicken Zoodle Soup, 67
    Easy Beef Stew with Carrot
      and Sweet Potato, 78
    Green Minestrone, 68
    Hearty Pot Roast, 93
    Quick Beef Pho, 97
    Savory Sausage Bread
      Pudding, 26
    Stuffed Cabbage Soup, 94
    Sweet Potato Chowder, 69
    Sweet Potato Shepherd's
      Pie, 85
    Tortilla-less Green Chicken
      Enchiladas, 74
    Whole Chicken with Pearl
      Onions, 82
organic foods, 20

P

Pancakes, Jumbo Blueberry, 35
parsnips
    Mashed Sweet Potatoes, 111
    Parsnip Soup, 64
    Root Vegetable Soup, 101

pies
    Crustless Sweet Potato Pie,
      142
    Sweet Potato Shepherd's
      Pie, 85
poblano peppers: Tortilla-less
  Green Chicken Enchiladas, 74
pork
    Melt-in-Your-Mouth Carnitas,
      90
    No-Wrap Pork Dumplings,
      47
    Pork and Collard Greens, 86
    Pork Chops with Cherry
      Sauce, 81
Porridge, Nut and Seed, 30
potatoes
    See also sweet potatoes
    Fondant Potatoes, 105
Pot Roast, Hearty, 93
pudding
    Coconut Chia Pudding, 133
    Soothing Tapioca Pudding,
      153
    Sticky Ginger Pudding, 154
pumpkin seeds: Nut and Seed
  Porridge, 30

Q

quercetin, 35, 36, 48, 60, 81, 86,
  89, 90, 107, 112, 115, 116, 125,
  129, 146, 161

R

radishes
    Breakfast Hash, 22
    Ground Turkey Taco Bowls,
      43
Ribs with Gravy, Braised Short,
  89
Roast, Hearty Pot, 93
Root Vegetable Soup, 101
rutabaga: Root Vegetable
  Soup, 101

S

salads
    Almost Niçoise Salad, 55
    Anti-Inflammatory Egg
      Salad, 137
    Broccoli Salad, 56
    Gingery Chicken Salad, 52
    Power Veggie Bowl with
      Carrot-Ginger Dressing, 51
sausage
    Sausage and Kale Stew, 77
    Savory Sausage Bread
      Pudding, 26
scallions
    Anti-Inflammatory Egg
      Salad, 137
    Gingery Chicken Salad, 52
    No-Wrap Pork Dumplings,
      47
    Scallion Egg Bites, 33
seeds. See nuts and seeds
sesame seeds
    Nut and Seed Porridge, 30
    Sesame Cabbage, 116
shallots
    Creamy Cauliflower Soup,
      60
    Honey-Shallot Vinaigrette,
      55
    Lamb Shanks with Shallots,
      73
Shepherd's Pie, Sweet Potato,
  85
shopping tips, 20
side dishes
    Braised Kale, 106
    Brown Butter Asparagus, 120
    Coconut Cauliflower Rice,
      107
    Fondant Potatoes, 105
    Garlic Mashed Cauliflower,
      112
    Glazed Carrots, 102
    Honey Beets, 108
    Mashed Sweet Potatoes, 111
    Mini Cauliflower Patties, 115
    Sesame Cabbage, 116
    Steamed Artichokes with
      Garlic Butter, 119

Steamed Sweet Potato, 126
Whole Herby Cauliflower, 125
Zoodles with Herb Butter, 123
Zucchini Medallions, 124
snacks
    Antihistamine Artichoke Dip, 138
    Anti-Inflammatory Egg Salad, 137
    Caramelized Onion Dip, 141
    Cauliflower Hummus, 129
    Coconut Chia Pudding, 133
    Large Batch Golden Turmeric Milk, 130
    prepping, 20
soups
    Asparagus and Dill Soup, 59
    Chicken Zoodle Soup, 67
    Creamy Cauliflower Soup, 60
    Green Minestrone, 68
    Healing Chicken Soup with Ginger and Turmeric, 98
    Parsnip Soup, 64
    Quick Beef Pho, 97
    Root Vegetable Soup, 101
    Stuffed Cabbage Soup, 94
    Sweet Potato Chowder, 69
    Thai-Style Carrot Soup, 63
stews
    Easy Beef Stew with Carrot and Sweet Potato, 78
    Sausage and Kale Stew, 77
sunflower seeds
    Nut and Seed Porridge, 30
    Sunflower Seed Queso, 134
sweet bread: Mini Blueberry Loaf, 36
sweet potatoes
    Breakfast Hash, 22
    Crustless Sweet Potato Pie, 142
    Easy Beef Stew with Carrot and Sweet Potato, 78
    Mashed Sweet Potatoes, 111

Power Veggie Bowl with Carrot-Ginger Dressing, 51
Steamed Sweet Potato, 126
Sunflower Seed Queso, 134
Sweet Potato Chowder, 69
Sweet Potato Shepherd's Pie, 85
Swiss chard
    Antihistamine Artichoke Dip, 138
    Egg Cups with Mixed Greens, 29
    Savory Sausage Bread Pudding, 26

T
Taco Bowls, Ground Turkey, 43
Tapioca Pudding, Soothing, 153
tigernut flour
    Cherry Apple Crumble, 161
    Jumbo Blueberry Pancakes, 35
    Maple Blondies, 149
    Mini Blueberry Loaf, 36
    Sticky Ginger Pudding, 154
    Upside-Down Apple Cake, 145
tortillas: Melt-in-Your-Mouth Carnitas, 90
turkey
    Ground Turkey Taco Bowls, 43
    Savory Sausage Bread Pudding, 26
turmeric
    Healing Chicken Soup with Ginger and Turmeric, 98
    Large Batch Golden Turmeric Milk, 130
turnips: Hearty Pot Roast, 93

V
vegetables
    See also specific types
    portioning, 21

W
white blood cells, 11

Z
zucchini
    Chicken Zoodle Soup, 67
    Green Minestrone, 68
    Tortilla-less Green Chicken Enchiladas, 74
    Zoodles with Herb Butter, 123
    Zucchini Medallions, 124